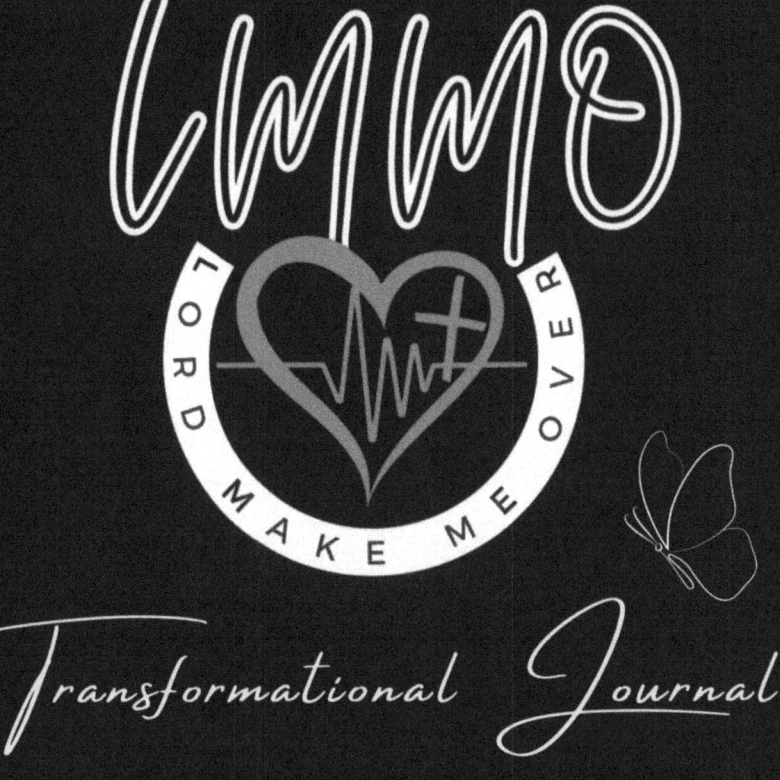

LMMO

LORD MAKE ME OVER

Transformational Journal

"GETTING TO THE HEART OF THE MATTER"

A 12 MONTH JOURNEY TO HELP YOU WALK IN THE FULLNESS OF YOUR PURPOSE BY EQUIPPING, EDUCATING AND EMPOWERING YOU TO REACH YOUR FULL TRANSFORMATION IN CHRIST.

LMMO
Lord Make Me Over
Transformational Journal
Getting to the Heart of the Matter

Published by
Kingdom Publishing, LLC
Odenton, MD

First printed in the USA

Copyright ©2026 Rhonda Sneed

ISBN: 978-1-967006-16-8

LORD MAKE ME OVER
TRANSFORMATIONAL *Journal*

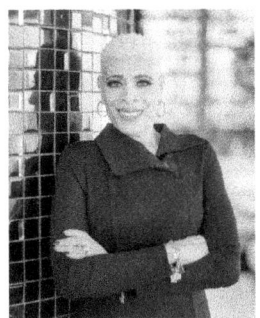

A Letter From The Purpose Pusher...

Dear Beloved,

I hope this letter finds you well and full of peace. In the busyness of our daily lives, it's easy to forget the importance of walking in purpose and the incredible call we have to devote ourselves to God. I want to encourage you, to use this transformational journal to pause and reflect on the deep, meaningful spiritual journey ahead of you—the one where each step can be a step of purpose, each moment an opportunity to draw closer to God. Our lives are not random or without direction. God has a plan for each of us, one uniquely designed with intention. When we commit to walking with Him, we allow that plan to unfold with grace and wisdom. You are not here by accident. Every gift you have, every challenge you face, every relationship you build there is purpose woven through all of it. It's easy to feel lost, overwhelmed, or unsure. But even in those moments, God calls us to trust in His guidance. To walk in purpose means to walk with faith and trust knowing that He will direct our steps, even when the path ahead isn't clear. Devote yourself to His will, and you will find peace, strength, and clarity that transcend understanding. Walking in purpose doesn't mean we won't face difficulties or moments of doubt, but it means we know we are never alone. God is always with us, guiding, providing, and carrying us. It is His strength, not our own, that will sustain us. So, I encourage you to seek Him daily, commit to staying focused on your spiritual growth, making time for prayer, for reflection, and for listening. Let your heart be open to His whispers. Know that when you devote yourself to Him, you are stepping into the purpose He has set for you, one that is infinitely more fulfilling than anything we could plan on our own. Walk in purpose. Walk in faith. And trust that God will lead you every step of the way.

With peace, love and blessings,

Dr. Rhonda Sneed

Monthly
PLANNER

Month _____
PURPOSE

MON	TUE	WED	THU	FRI	SAT	SUN

I'm grateful for: --

Personal Testimonies:

Monthly Goal

◇ _____

◇ _____

◇ _____

PURPOSE

Scripture

"For we are God's masterpiece. He has created us anew in Christ Jesus, so we can do the good things he planned for us long ago."
Ephesians 2:10 NLT

Prayer

God as I come before You today, I humbly ask that You reveal to me the purpose You have designed for my life. Open my eyes to the unique gifts and talents You have given me, and guide me to use them to fulfill Your will for the Kingdom.

Affirmation

I will walk in the fullness of my purpose!

Spiritual Growth
MILESTONES

-
-
-

Reflection

- "How does this verse speak to your current life situation?"

- "What does this verse reveal about God's character?"

- How does my daily life align with the word **PURPOSE**!

Inspirational Quote

"You were created on purpose, with purpose, for purpose"!
~Dr. Rhonda Sneed

My mental health
Monthly Check In

Date _____

Mo   Tu   We   Th   Fr   Sa   Su

What brings you Joy?

How are you feeling this month?

_____

_____

_____

_____

_____

What did you worry about this month?

Am I satisfied with this month?

_____

_____

_____

_____

_____

How are you taking care of yourself?

Are you sleeping well?

_____

_____

_____

_____

_____

Habit Tracker

- ● Water
- ● Workout
- ● Take a walk
- ● Breathing exercises
- ● Meditation
- ● Read a book

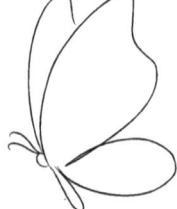

A Dose from Doc...

Purpose

You are uniquely designed for a purpose that only you can fulfill. Trust that God has equipped you with the gifts, strength, and courage to walk boldly in your purpose. Take one step at a time, knowing He is guiding you every step of the way. The kingdom needs what you have to offer go be great!

-Purpose Pusher-

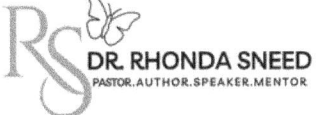

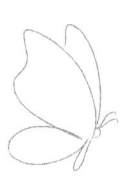

Monthly Acronym

USING EACH LETTER, DESCRIBE A TRANSFORMATIONAL EXPERIENCE

P _____

U _____

R _____

P _____

O _____

S _____

E _____

INSPIRATIONAL AFFIRMATIONS

Purpose

I am created with a unique purpose, and I trust that God is guiding me to fulfill it. (Ephesians 2:10)

God has a plan for my life, and I will walk in the purpose He has set before me. (Jeremiah 29:11)

I am committed to living each day with intention, knowing I am part of God's greater plan.

Every moment of my life has purpose, and I trust God to reveal it to me in His timing

I have everything I need to succeed within me.

Choose or create affirmations that resonates deeply with you and reflects the mindset or attitude you wish to embody throughout your day. Repeat it to yourself as part of your morning routine, perhaps during meditation, while getting ready, or whenever it feels most effective for you. This repetition can help focus your mind and set a positive intention for the day ahead.

notes

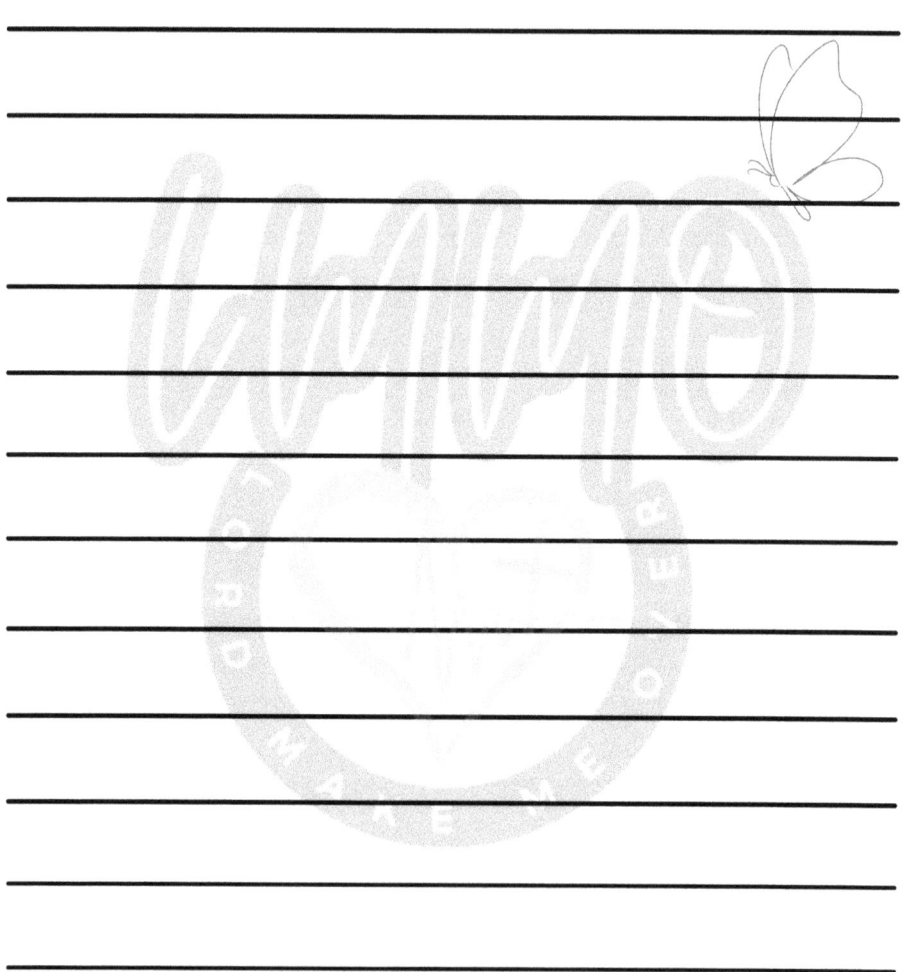

notes

notes

notes

notes

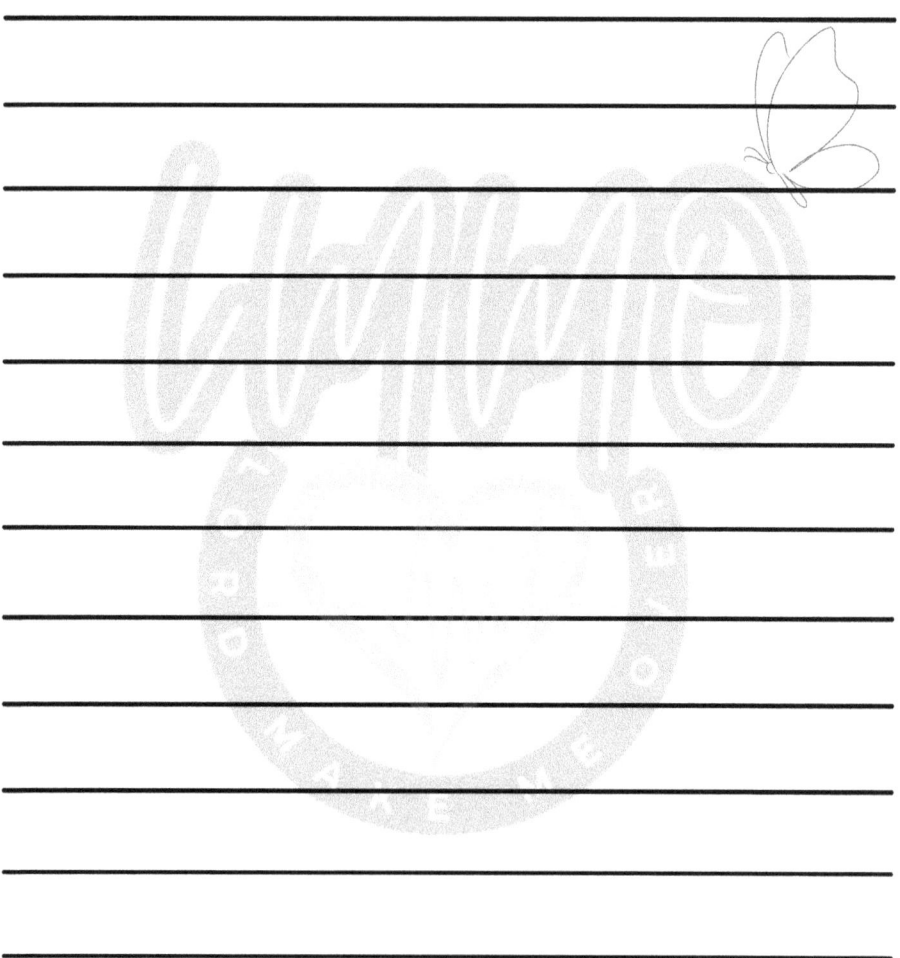

notes

_____

_____

_____

_____

_____

_____

_____

_____

_____

Monthly
PLANNER

Month _____

BELIEVE

MON	TUE	WED	THU	FRI	SAT	SUN

I'm grateful for: --

Personal Testimonies:

Monthly Goal

◇ _____

◇ _____

◇ _____

BELIEVE

Scripture

"Jesus said to him, "If you can believe, all things are possible to him who believes."
Mark 9:23 NKJV

Prayer

God, help me to see my circumstances as opportunities for spiritual growth. And help me to make daily decisions to believe in your word no matter what I may face.

Affirmation

I will believe God with all of my heart.

Spiritual Growth
MILESTONES

-
-
-

Reflection

- "How does this verse speak to your current life situation?"

- "What does this verse reveal about God's character?"

- How does my daily life align with the word **BELIEVE**!

Inspirational Quote

"In order to succeed, we must first believe that we can."
~ Nikos Kazantzakis

My mental health
Monthly Check In

Date _____

Mo   Tu   We   Th   Fr   Sa   Su

What brings you Joy?

_____

_____

_____

How are you feeling this month?

😍 😊 😐 😣 😞

_____

What did you worry about this month?

_____

_____

_____

Am I satisfied with this month?

😍 😊 😐 😣 😞

_____

How are you taking care of yourself?

_____

_____

_____

Are you sleeping well?

😍 😊 😐 😣 😞

_____

Habit Tracker

⬤ Water
⬤ Workout
⬤ Take a walk
⬤ Breathing exercises
⬤ Meditation
⬤ Read a book

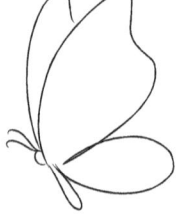

A Dose from Doc...

Believe

Trust in God with all your heart, knowing He is faithful and His plans for you are good. Even when the path seems unclear, His love never fails, and His promises are true. Surrender your worries, and let His peace guide you. He's with you every step of the way—believe it fully!

-Purpose Pusher-

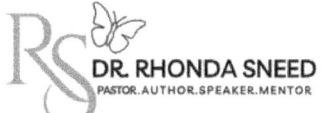

DR. RHONDA SNEED
PASTOR.AUTHOR.SPEAKER.MENTOR

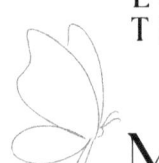

Monthly Acronym

USING EACH LETTER, DESCRIBE A
TRANSFORMATIONAL EXPERIENCE

B _____

E _____

L _____

I _____

E _____

V _____

E _____

INSPIRATIONAL AFFIRMATIONS

Believe

I believe that with God, all things are possible. (Matthew 19:26)

I believe in God's promises, and I trust He will fulfill them in my life.

I believe that God is working everything for my good, even when I can't see it. (Romans 8:28)

I believe that faith as small as a mustard seed can move mountains. (Matthew 17:20)

I believe I am enough.

Choose or create affirmations that resonates deeply with you and reflects the mindset or attitude you wish to embody throughout your day. Repeat it to yourself as part of your morning routine, perhaps during meditation, while getting ready, or whenever it feels most effective for you. This repetition can help focus your mind and set a positive intention for the day ahead.

Monthly
PLANNER

Month _____

TRUST

MON	TUE	WED	THU	FRI	SAT	SUN

I'm grateful for: --

Personal Testimonies:

Monthly Goal
◇ _____
◇ _____
◇ _____

TRUST

Scripture

"Trust in the Lord with all your heart, And lean not on your own understanding; In all your ways acknowledge Him, And He shall direct your paths."
Proverbs 3:5-6 NKJV

Prayer

God, help me trust you with my decisions and future. Let me lean on you with all my heart instead of relying on my own imperfect understanding.

Affirmation

I will trust God with all of me.

Spiritual Growth
MILESTONES

-
-
-

Reflection

- "How does this verse speak to your current life situation?"

- "What does this verse reveal about God's character?"

- How does my daily life align with the word **TRUST**!

Inspirational Quote

"Trust is built with consistency".
~ Lincoln Chafee

My mental health
Monthly Check In

Date _____

What brings you Joy?

_____

_____

_____

How are you feeling this month?

😍 🙂 😐 😕 ☹️

_____

_____

What did you worry about this month?

_____

_____

_____

Am I satisfied with this month?

😍 🙂 😐 😕 ☹️

_____

_____

How are you taking care of yourself?

_____

_____

_____

Are you sleeping well?

😍 🙂 😐 😕 ☹️

_____

_____

Habit Tracker

● Water
● Workout
● Take a walk
● Breathing exercises
● Meditation
● Read a book

A Dose from Doc...

Trust

No matter what you're facing, trust that God is in control and working all things for your good. His timing is perfect, and His plans are greater than you can imagine. Lean on Him, and He will give you the strength and peace to keep moving forward. He is faithful—trust Him completely!

-Purpose Pusher-

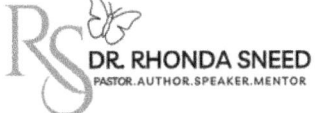

DR. RHONDA SNEED
PASTOR.AUTHOR.SPEAKER.MENTOR

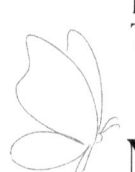

Monthly Acronym

USING EACH LETTER, DESCRIBE A
TRANSFORMATIONAL EXPERIENCE

T _____

R _____

U _____

S _____

T _____

INSPIRATIONAL AFFIRMATIONS
Trust

I trust in God's plan for me, even when I don't understand it.
(Proverbs 3:5-6)

God is my refuge, and I trust Him with every decision I make.
(Psalm 91:2)

I trust God to lead me, and I follow His guidance with faith
and confidence.

I trust God to provide for me in every area of my life.

I trust God with all of me.

Choose or create affirmations that resonates deeply with you and reflects the mindset or attitude you wish to embody throughout your day. Repeat it to yourself as part of your morning routine, perhaps during meditation, while getting ready, or whenever it feels most effective for you. This repetition can help focus your mind and set a positive intention for the day ahead.

notes

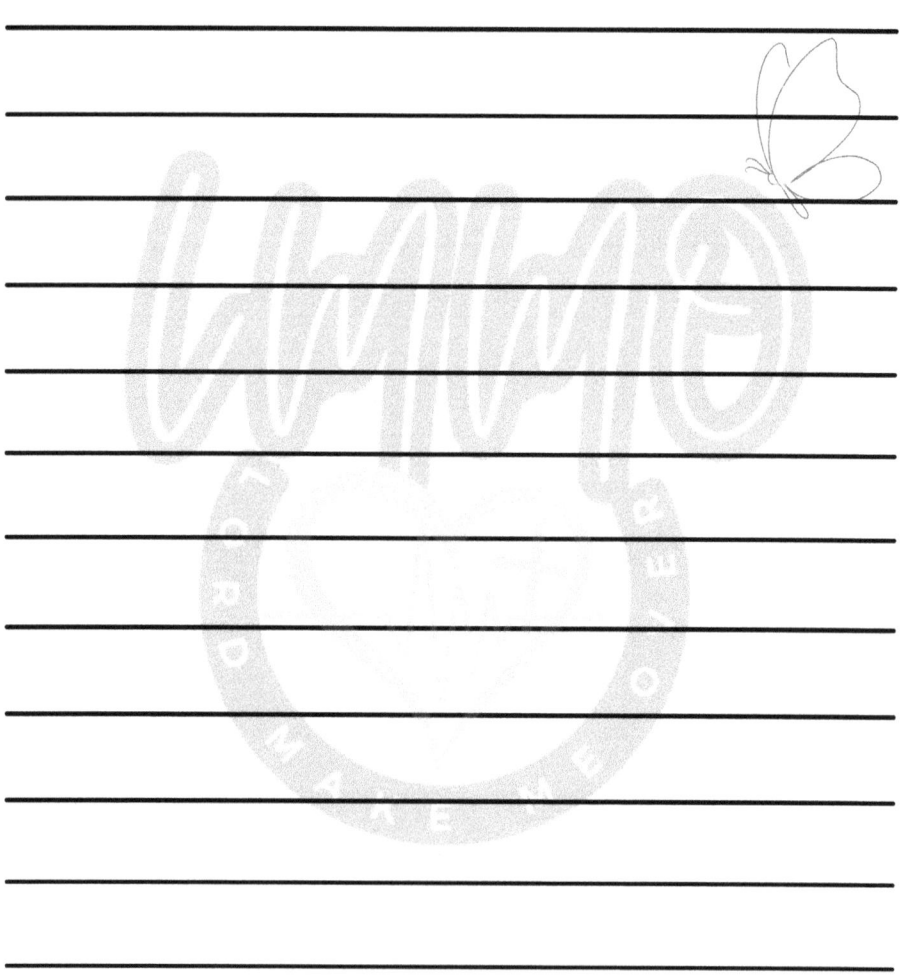

notes

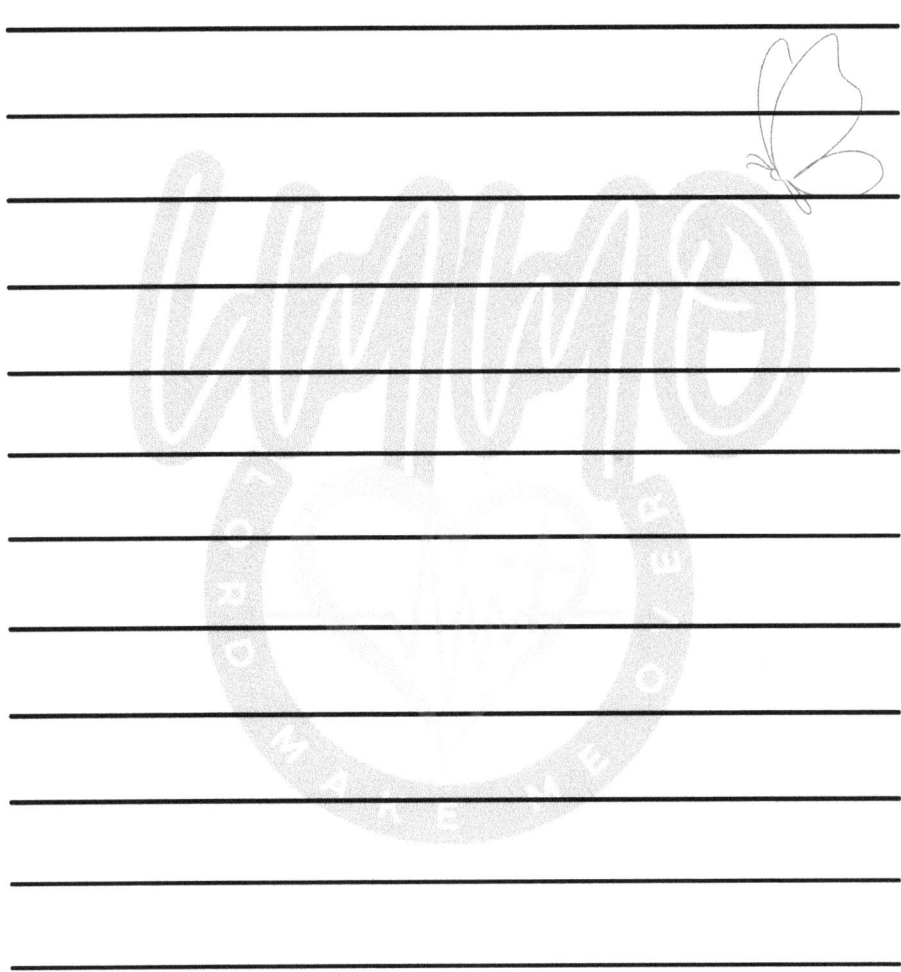

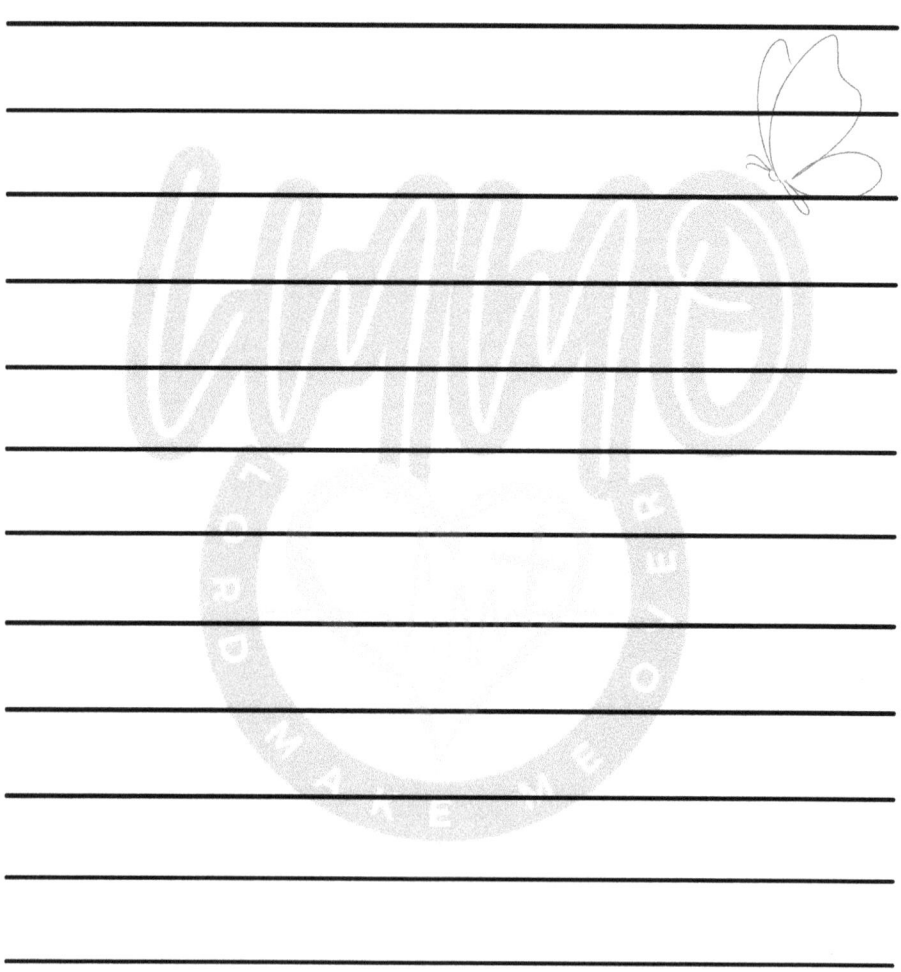

notes

_____

_____

_____

_____

_____

_____

_____

_____

_____

_____

_____

notes

_____

_____

_____

_____

_____

_____

_____

_____

_____

_____

notes

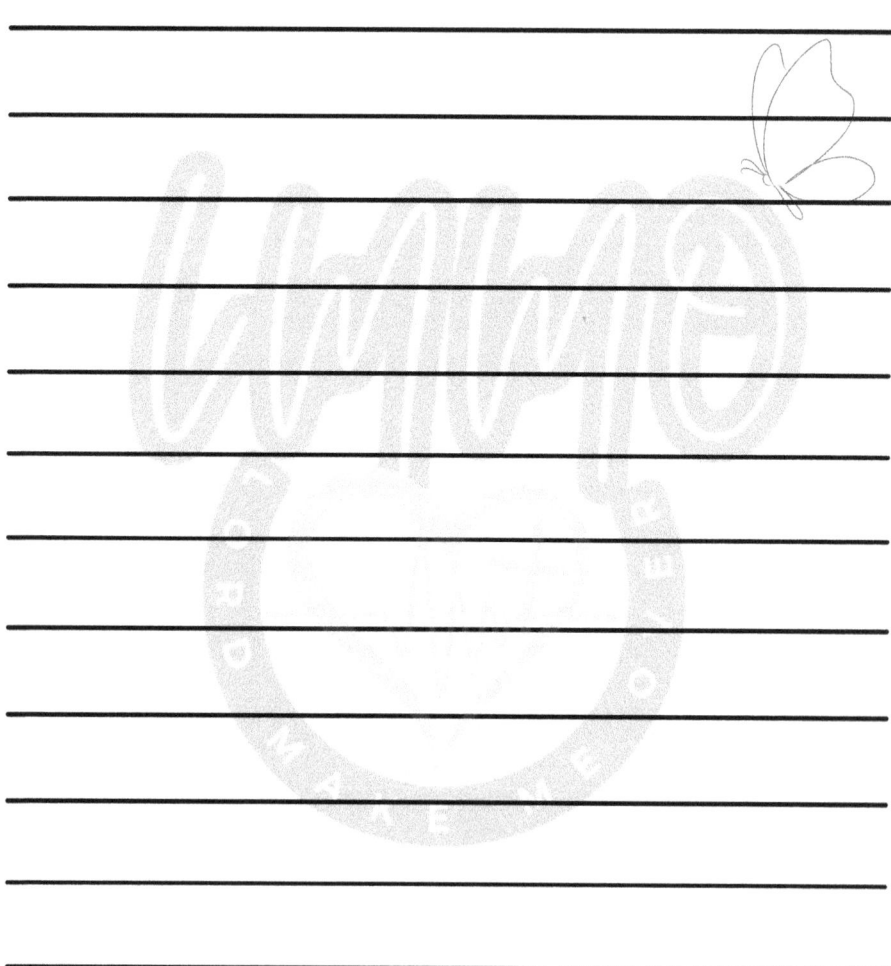

notes

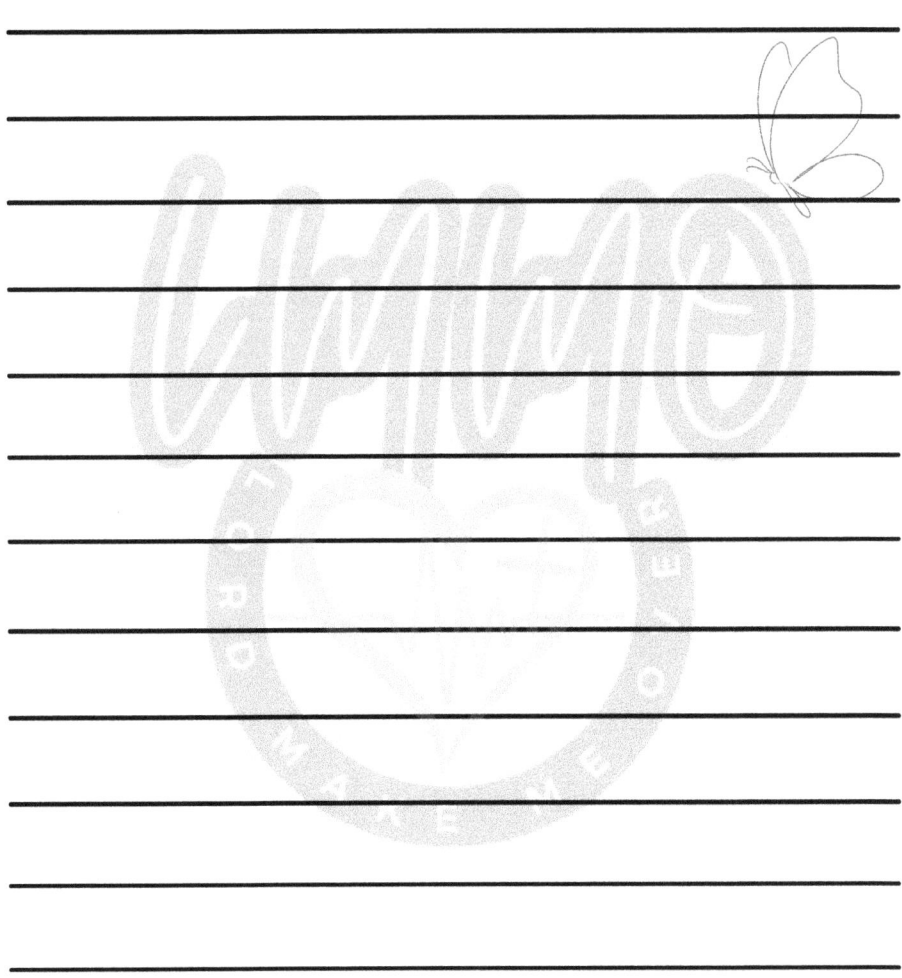

Monthly
PLANNER

Month _____

FAITH

MON	TUE	WED	THU	FRI	SAT	SUN

I'm grateful for: --

Personal Testimonies:

Monthly Goal

◇ _____

◇ _____

◇ _____

FAITH

Scripture

"But without faith it is impossible to please Him, for he who comes to God must believe that He is, and that He is a rewarder of those who diligently seek Him.
Hebrews 11:6 NKJV

Prayer

God, strengthen my faith in you today, help me to trust in your promises and guidance, even when I face challenges.

Affirmation

I will walk in unwavering faith.

Spiritual Growth
MILESTONES

-
-
-

Reflection

- "How does this verse speak to your current life situation?"

- "What does this verse reveal about God's character?"

- How does my daily life align with the word **FAITH**!

Inspirational Quote

"Faith is deliberate confidence in the character of God whose ways you may not understand at the time."
~ Oswald Chambers

My mental health
Monthly Check In

Date _____

Mo   Tu   We   Th   Fr   Sa   Su

What brings you Joy?

_____

_____

_____

How are you feeling this month?

😍 🙂 😐 😧 😫

_____

_____

What did you worry about this month?

_____

_____

_____

Am I satisfied with this month?

😍 🙂 😐 😧 😫

_____

_____

How are you taking care of yourself?

_____

_____

_____

Are you sleeping well?

😍 🙂 😐 😧 😫

_____

_____

Habit Tracker

- ● Water
- ● Workout
- ● Take a walk
- ● Breathing exercises
- ● Meditation
- ● Read a book

A Dose from Doc...

Faith

Keep your faith in God strong, even when things seem uncertain. He sees the bigger picture and is working everything out for your good. Trust His love, His promises, and His perfect timing. With faith, things can change for the better, and your heart can find peace. Hold on—He's got you!

-Purpose Pusher-

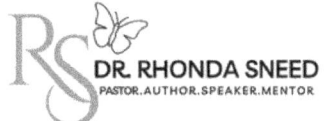

DR. RHONDA SNEED
PASTOR.AUTHOR.SPEAKER.MENTOR

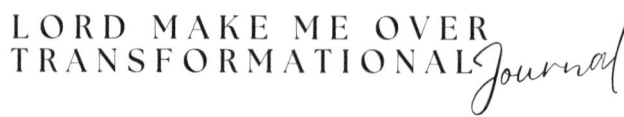

Monthly Acronym

USING EACH LETTER, DESCRIBE A
TRANSFORMATIONAL EXPERIENCE

F _____

A _____

I _____

T _____

H _____

INSPIRATIONAL
AFFIRMATIONS
Faith

I walk by faith, not by sight, trusting God in every season of my life.
(2 Corinthians 5:7)

My faith is unwavering because I know that God is faithful.

With faith in God, I can overcome any obstacle that comes my way.
(Mark 11:22-24)

I trust in God's power to strengthen and equip me for whatever I face.

I trust God to provide for me daily.

Choose or create affirmations that resonates deeply with you and reflects the mindset or attitude you wish to embody throughout your day. Repeat it to yourself as part of your morning routine, perhaps during meditation, while getting ready, or whenever it feels most effective for you. This repetition can help focus your mind and set a positive intention for the day ahead.

notes

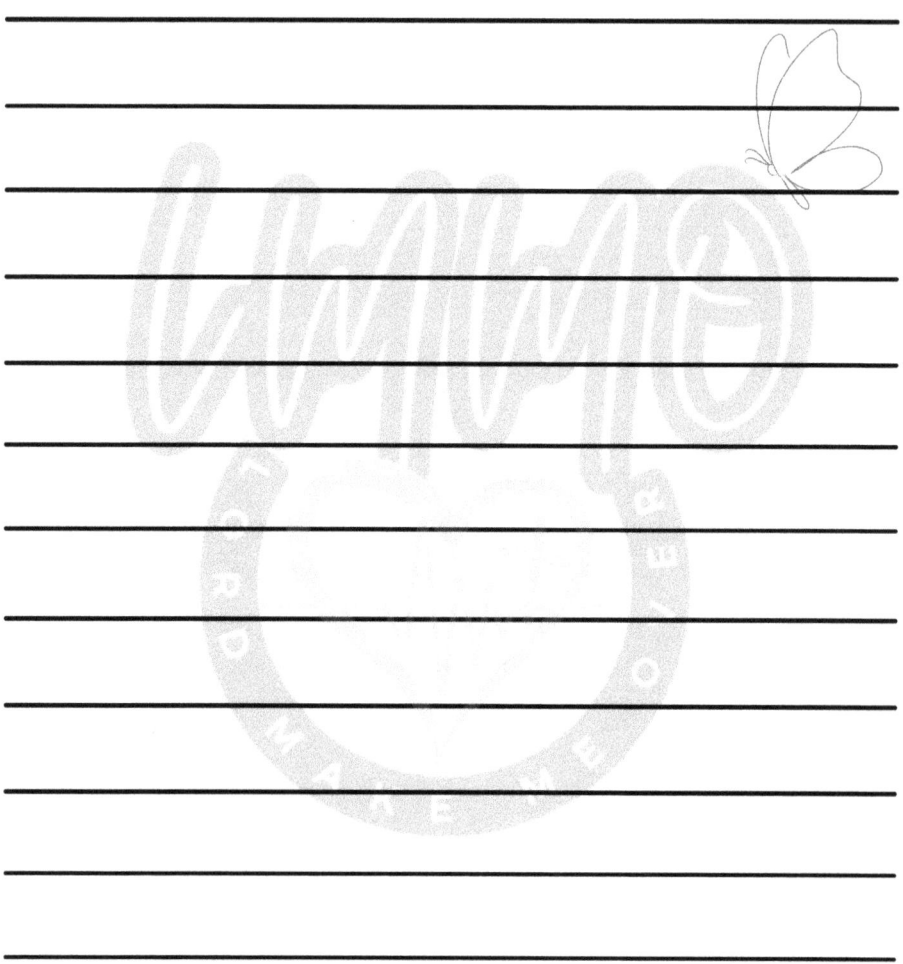

_____

_____

_____

_____

_____

_____

_____

_____

_____

_____

notes

notes

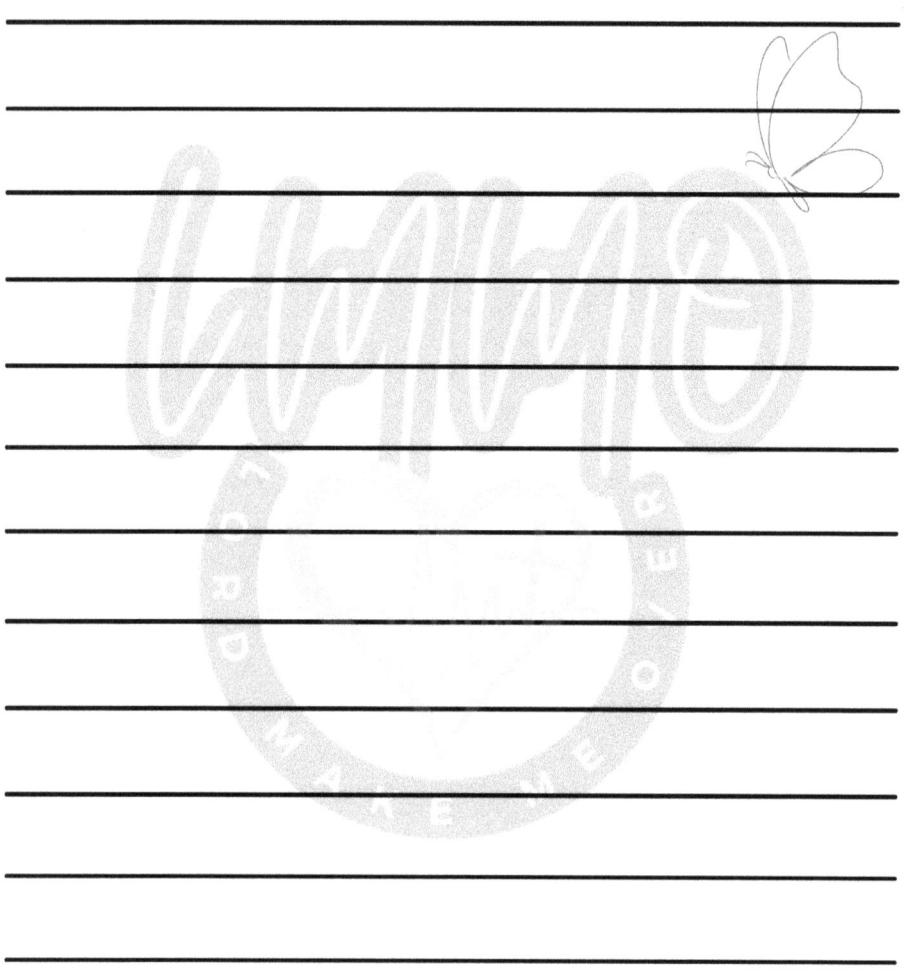

notes

notes

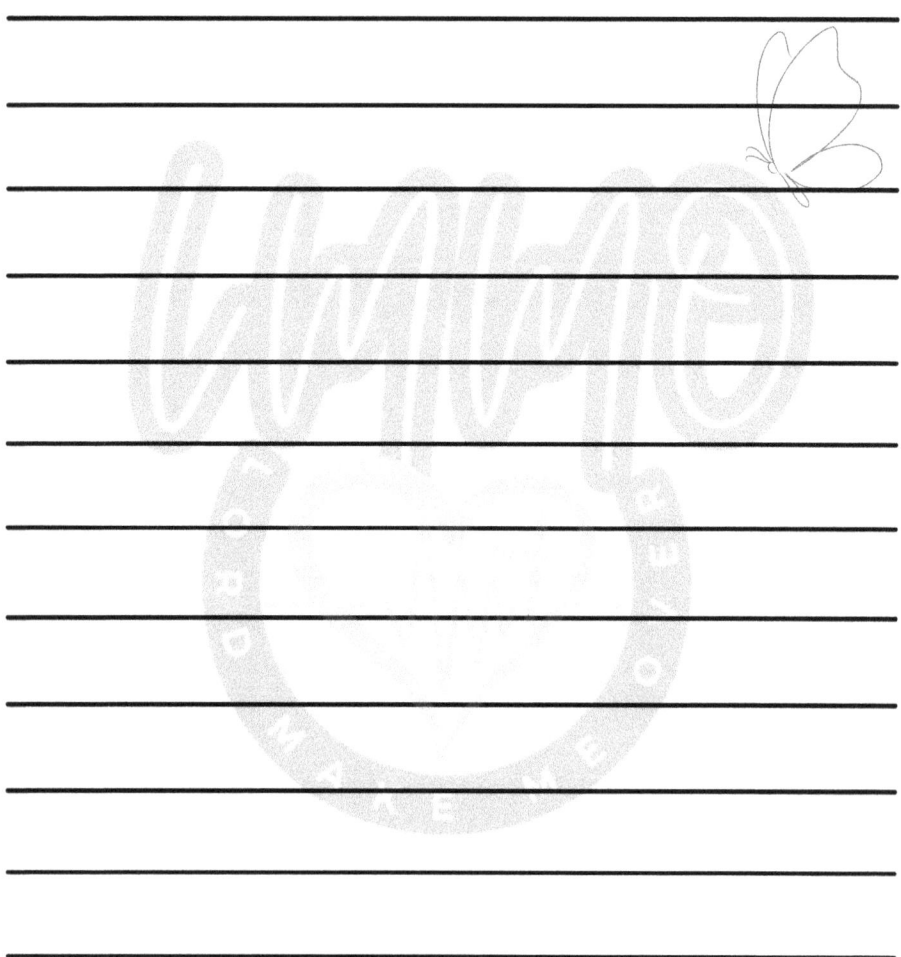

notes

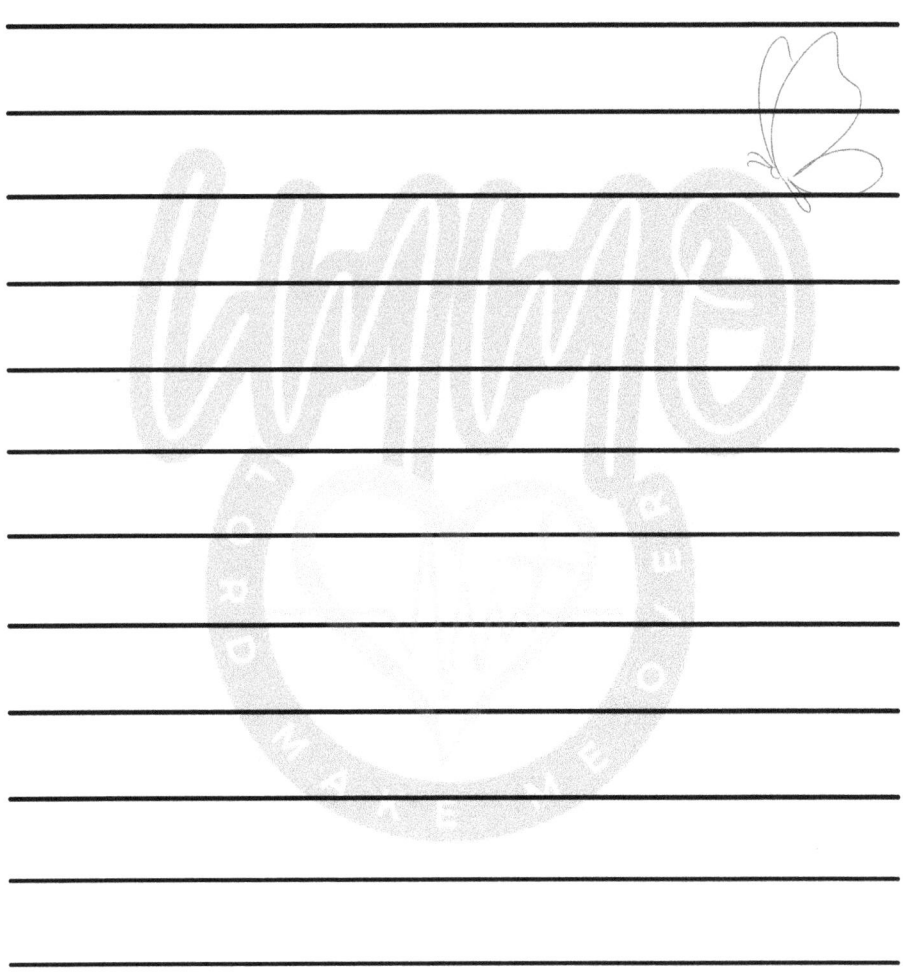

_____

_____

_____

_____

_____

_____

_____

_____

_____

_____

_____

Monthly
PLANNER

Month _____

LOVE

MON	TUE	WED	THU	FRI	SAT	SUN

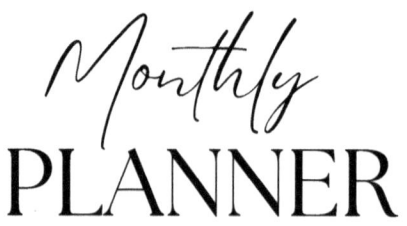

I'm grateful for: --

Personal Testimonies:

Monthly Goal

◇ _____

◇ _____

◇ _____

LOVE

Scripture

"But you, O Lord, are a God of compassion and mercy, slow to get angry and filled with unfailing love and faithfulness."
Psalms 86:15 NLT

Prayer

God, bless us with Love, that we may Love as you Love! That we may show patience, tolerance, kindness, care and love to all.

Affirmation

I will demonstrate the LOVE of Christ.

Spiritual Growth

MILESTONES

-
-
-

Reflection

- "How does this verse speak to your current life situation?"

- "What does this verse reveal about God's character?"

- How does my daily life align with the word **LOVE**!

Inspirational Quote

"**Spread love everywhere you go. Let no one ever come to you without leaving happier.**"
~ Mother Teresa

My mental health
Monthly Check In

Date _____

Mo   Tu   We   Th   Fr   Sa   Su

What brings you Joy?

_____

_____

_____

How are you feeling this month?

😍   🙂   😐   😖   ☹️

_____

What did you worry about this month?

_____

_____

_____

Am I satisfied with this month?

😍   🙂   😐   😖   ☹️

_____

How are you taking care of yourself?

_____

_____

_____

Are you sleeping well?

😍   🙂   😐   😖   ☹️

_____

Habit Tracker

- ⚫ Water
- ⚫ Workout
- ⚫ Take a walk
- ⚫ Breathing exercises
- ⚫ Meditation
- ⚫ Read a book

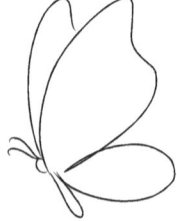

A Dose from Doc...

Love

Show the love of God by being kind, patient, and compassionate to those around you. Let your words uplift, your actions serve, and your heart reflect His grace. A simple act of kindness can shine His light in someone's life. Love without limits, just as He loves you!

-Purpose Pusher-

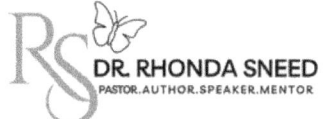

DR. RHONDA SNEED
PASTOR.AUTHOR.SPEAKER.MENTOR

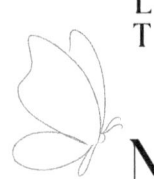

Monthly Acronym

USING EACH LETTER, DESCRIBE A TRANSFORMATIONAL EXPERIENCE

L _____

O _____

V _____

E _____

INSPIRATIONAL AFFIRMATIONS

Love

I am called to love others as Christ has loved me—unconditionally and without reservation. (John 13:34)

I choose to love even when it's hard, knowing that God is love and He empowers me to love others. (1 John 4:8)

Through God's love, I am transformed, and I am able to share that love with those around me.

God's love is the foundation of my life, and it guides my actions and decisions.

My mind is clear, my heart is open, and I am ready to embrace the day.

Choose or create affirmations that resonates deeply with you and reflects the mindset or attitude you wish to embody throughout your day. Repeat it to yourself as part of your morning routine, perhaps during meditation, while getting ready, or whenever it feels most effective for you. This repetition can help focus your mind and set a positive intention for the day ahead.

notes

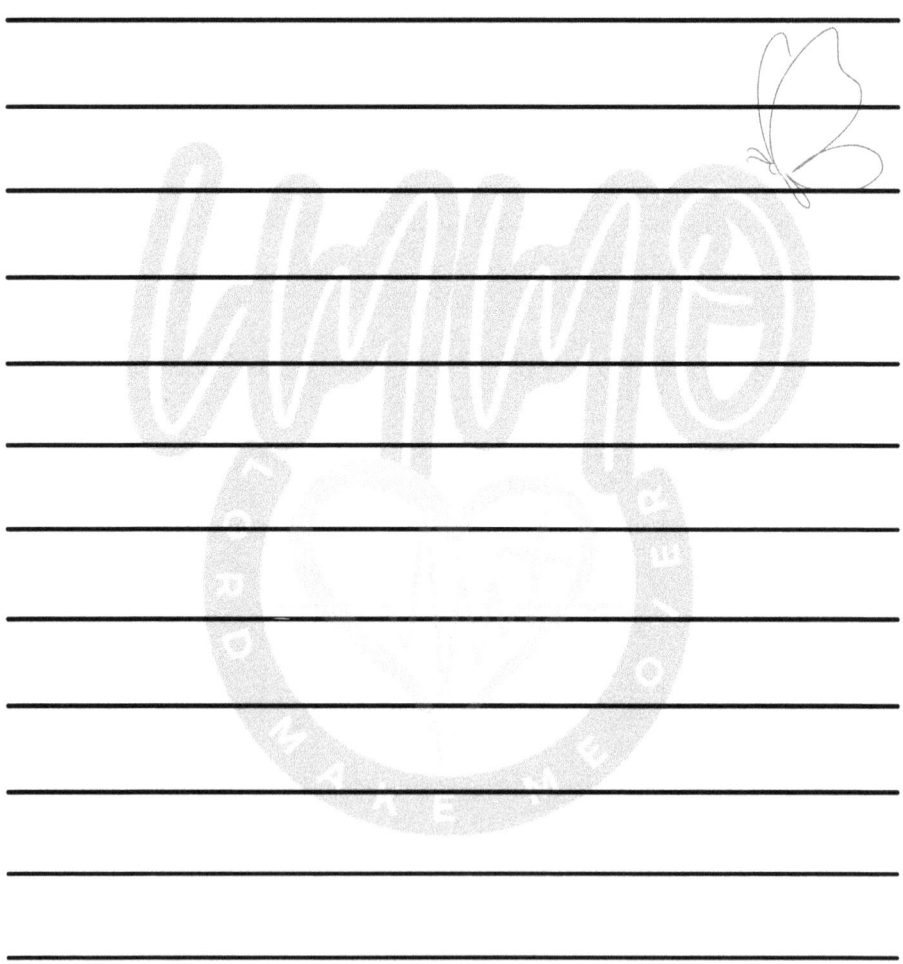

_____

_____

_____

_____

_____

_____

_____

_____

_____

_____

notes

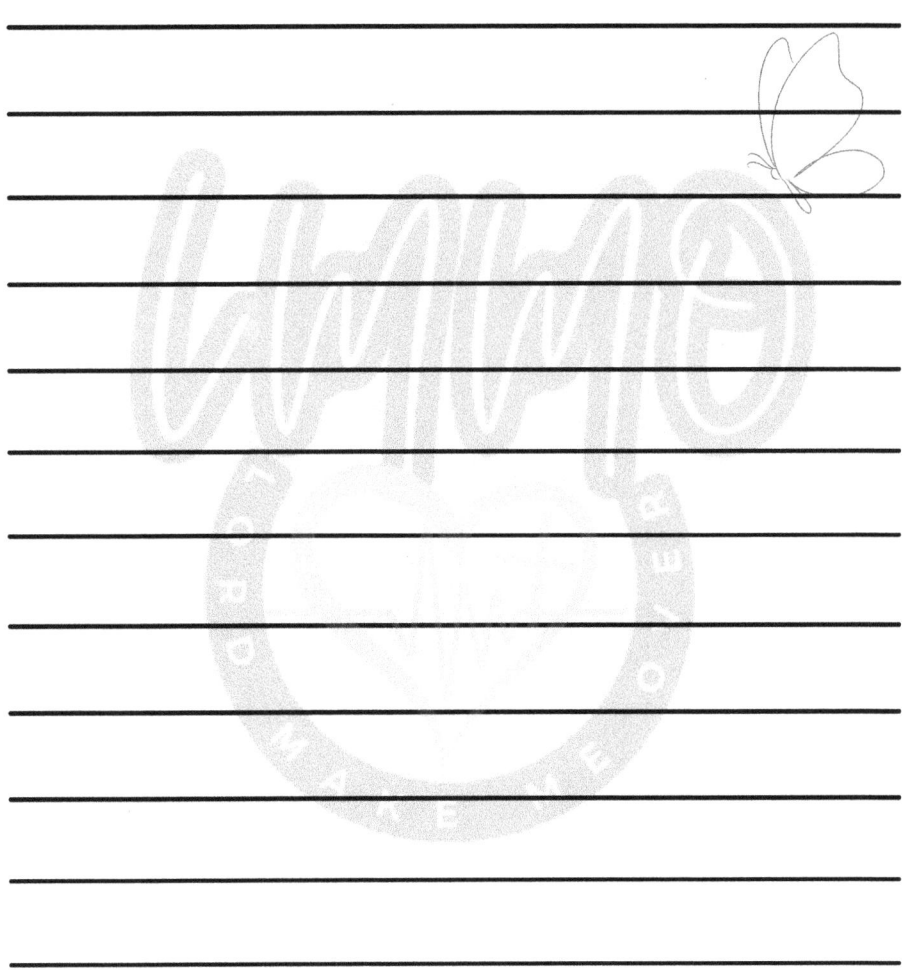

notes

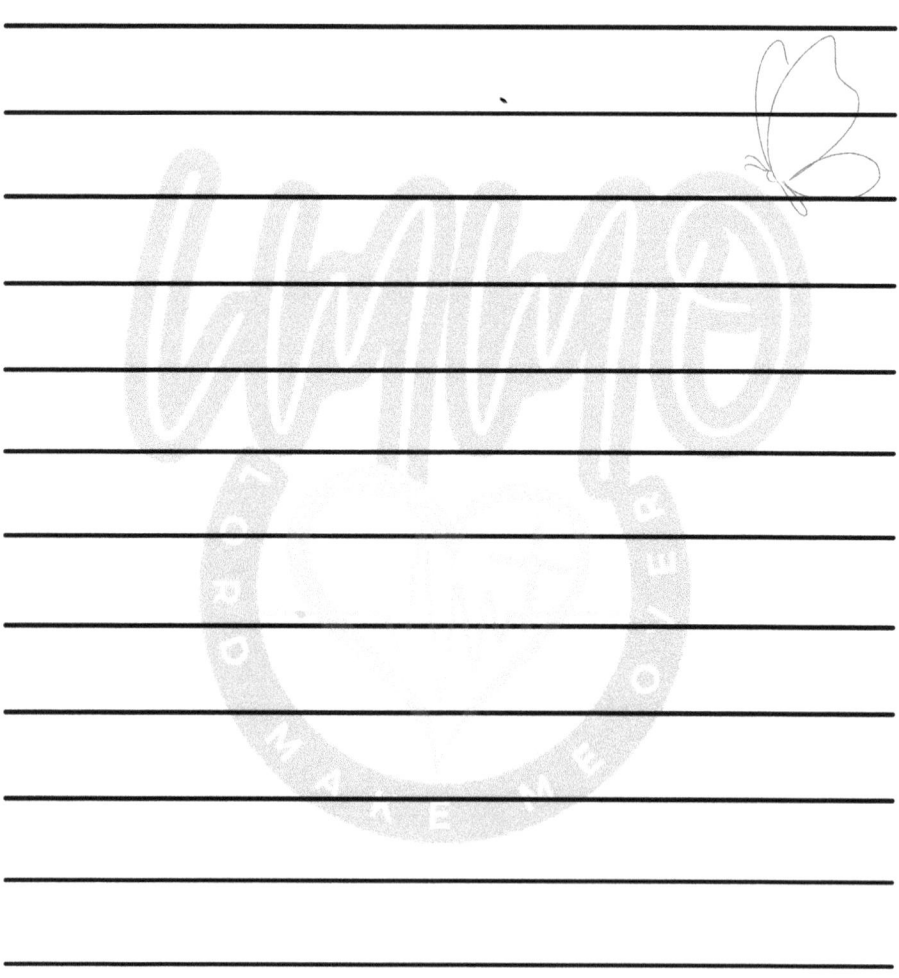

notes

notes

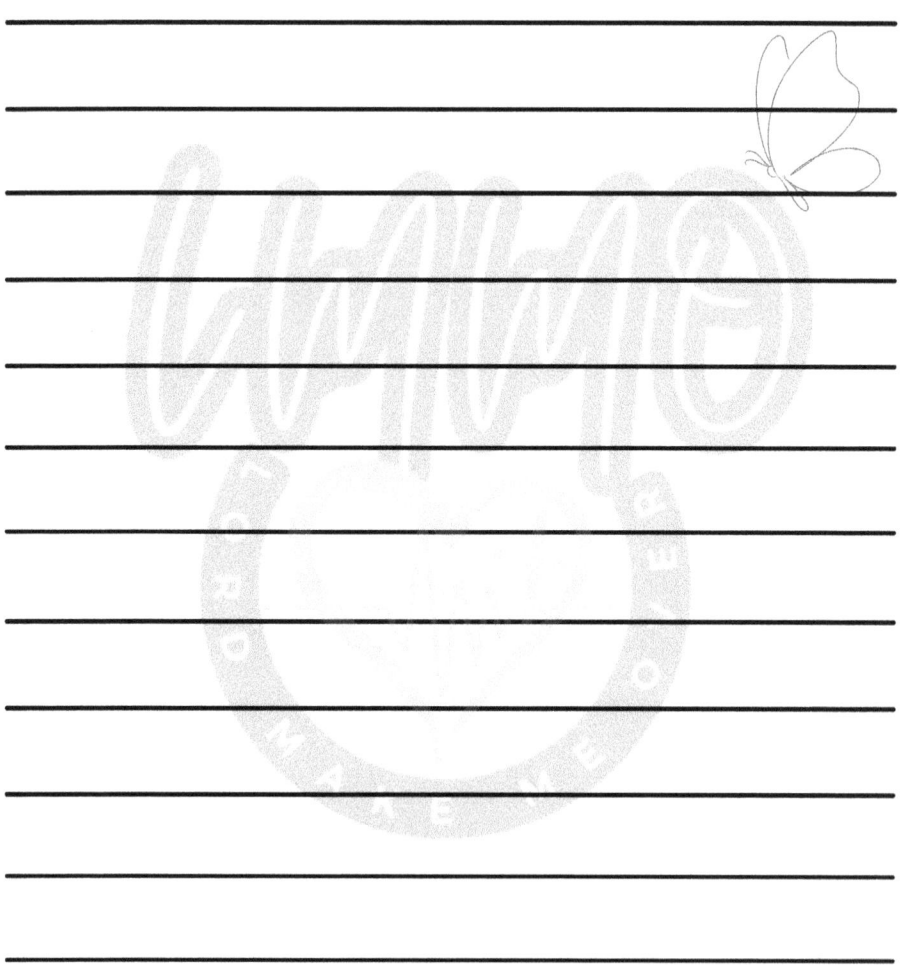

---

notes

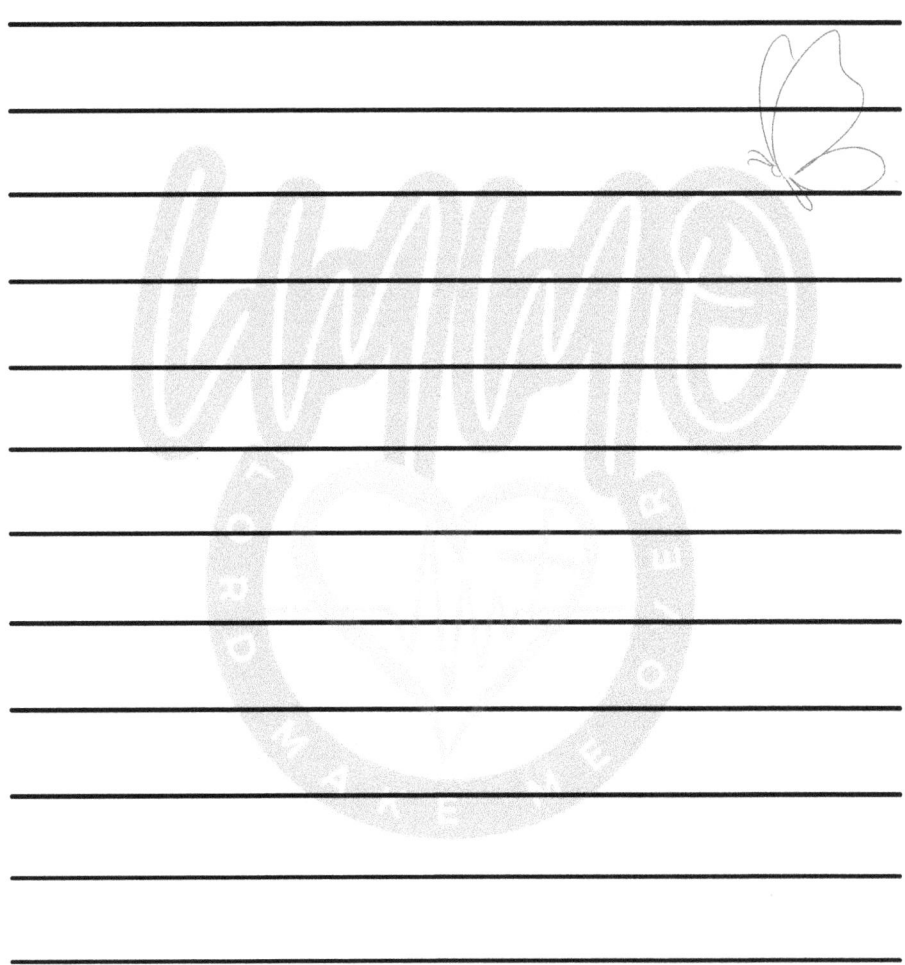

Monthly PLANNER

Month _____

TRANSFORMATION

MON	TUE	WED	THU	FRI	SAT	SUN

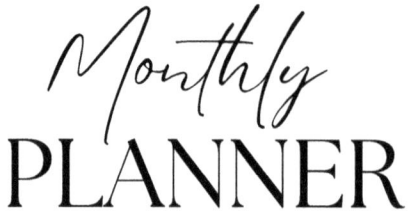

I'm grateful for: _____

_____

Personal Testimonies:

Monthly Goal

◇ _____

◇ _____

◇ _____

TRANSFORMATION

Scripture

"Don't copy the behavior and customs of this world, but let God transform you into a new person by changing the way you think. Then you will learn to know God's will for you, which is good and pleasing and perfect."
Romans 12:2 NLT

Prayer

God, I receive Your transforming, restoring, and renewing power in my life today. I declare that I am a new creature in Christ Jesus, and I am beginning anew with You today.

Affirmation

My mind is transformed daily.

Spiritual Growth
MILESTONES

-
-
-

Reflection

- "How does this verse speak to your current life situation?"

- "What does this verse reveal about God's character?"

- How does my daily life align with the word **TRANSFORMATION**!

Inspirational Quote

"It's time to SHIFT-Stepping, Higher, Into, Full, Transformation Trusting God"
-Dr. Rhonda Sneed

My mental health
Monthly Check In

Date _____

Mo   Tu   We   Th   Fr   Sa   Su

What brings you Joy?

_____

_____

_____

How are you feeling this month?

😍 🙂 😐 😟 😣

_____

What did you worry about this month?

_____

_____

_____

Am I satisfied with this month?

😍 🙂 😐 😟 😣

_____

How are you taking care of yourself?

_____

_____

_____

Are you sleeping well?

😍 🙂 😐 😟 😣

_____

Habit Tracker

- ⬤ Water
- ⬤ Workout
- ⬤ Take a walk
- ⬤ Breathing exercises
- ⬤ Meditation
- ⬤ Read a book

A Dose from Doc...

Transformation

Let God transform your life by surrendering everything to Him—your fears, struggles, and plans. Spend time in His Word, seek Him in prayer, and trust His work in your heart. Transformation takes time, but with God, you'll become the masterpiece He created you to be. Stay open and watch Him work wonders!

-Purpose Pusher-

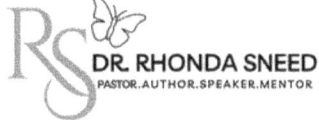

DR. RHONDA SNEED
PASTOR.AUTHOR.SPEAKER.MENTOR

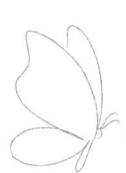

LORD MAKE ME OVER
TRANSFORMATIONAL *Journal*

Monthly Acronym

USING EACH LETTER, DESCRIBE A
TRANSFORMATIONAL EXPERIENCE

T _____

R _____

A _____

N _____

S _____

F _____

O _____

R _____

M _____

INSPIRATIONAL
AFFIRMATIONS
Transformation

I am being transformed daily by the renewing of my mind through God's Word. (Romans 12:2)

God is working in me, making me more like Christ each day.

I embrace the process of transformation, trusting that God's work in me is for my good.

I am not the same person I used to be; I am a new creation in Christ. (2 Corinthians 5:17)

I am not defined by my past; I am driven by my future.

Choose or create affirmations that resonates deeply with you and reflects the mindset or attitude you wish to embody throughout your day. Repeat it to yourself as part of your morning routine, perhaps during meditation, while getting ready, or whenever it feels most effective for you. This repetition can help focus your mind and set a positive intention for the day ahead.

notes

notes

_____

_____

_____

_____

_____

_____

_____

_____

_____

_____

_____

notes

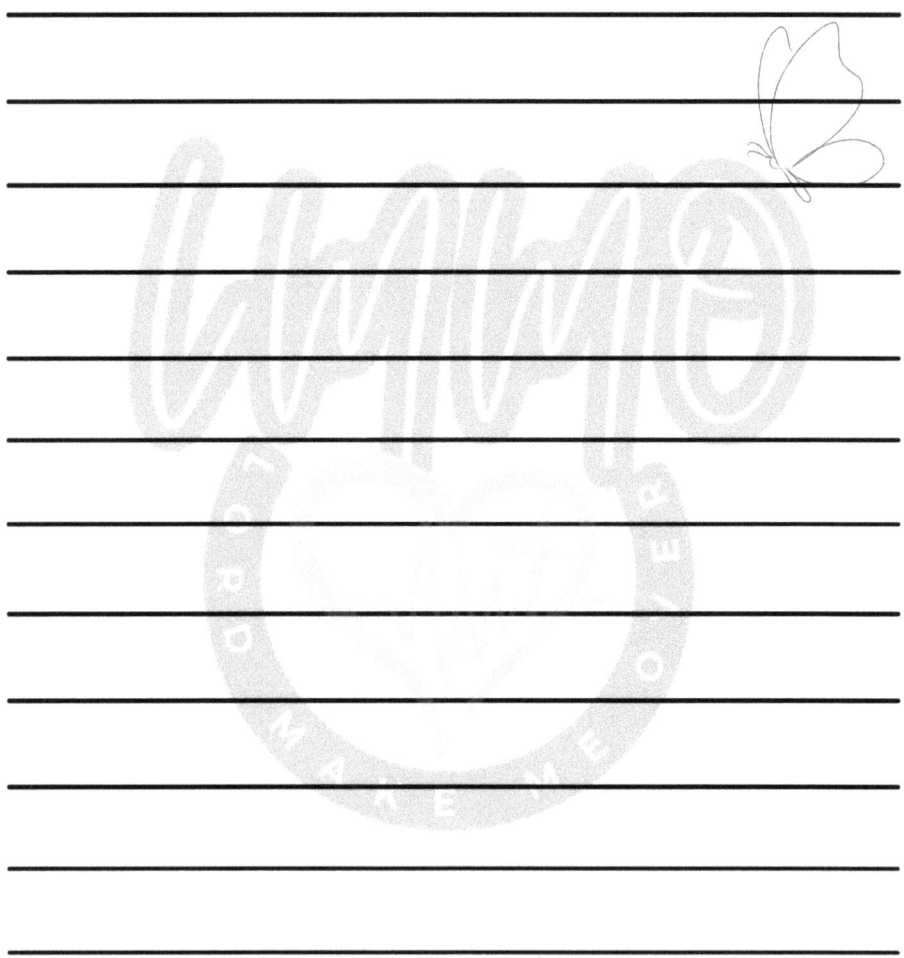

_____

_____

_____

_____

_____

_____

_____

_____

_____

_____

notes

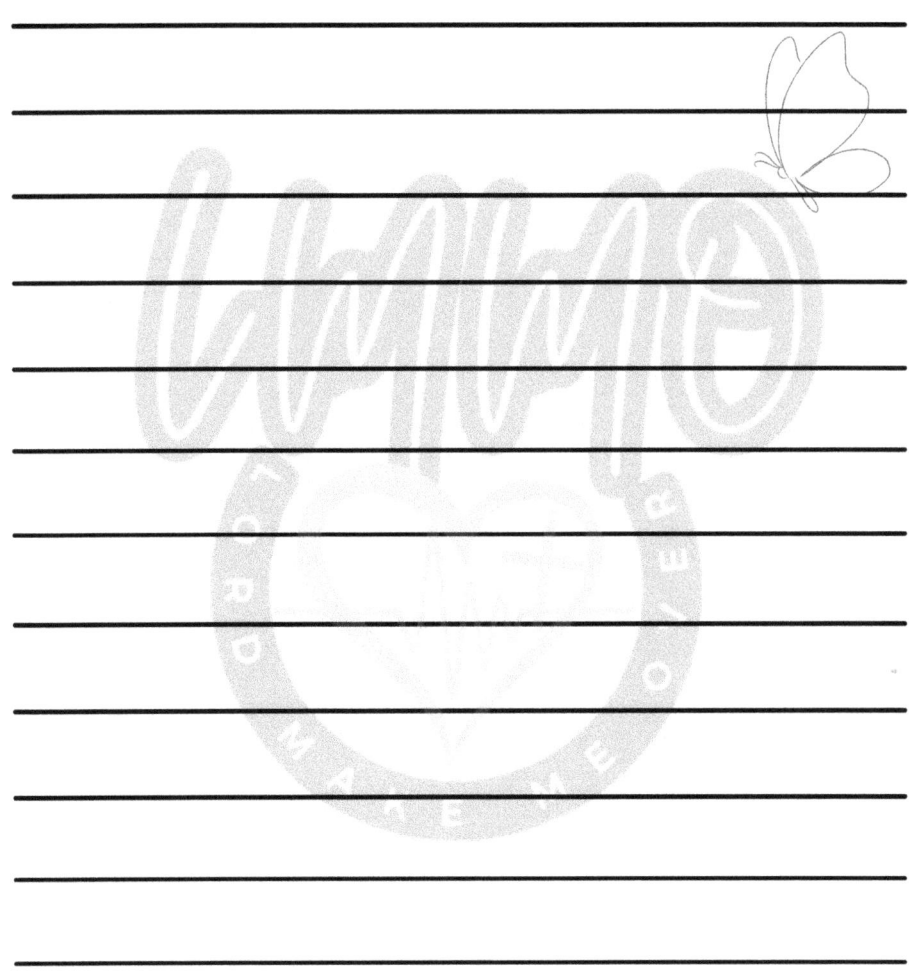

notes

_____

_____

_____

_____

_____

_____

_____

_____

_____

_____

notes

_____

_____

_____

_____

_____

_____

_____

_____

_____

_____

Monthly
PLANNER

Month _____

GRATITUDE

MON	TUE	WED	THU	FRI	SAT	SUN

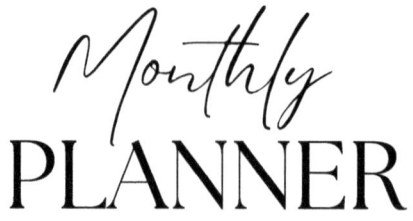

I'm grateful for: --

Personal Testimonies:

Monthly Goal

◇ _____

◇ _____

◇ _____

GRATITUDE

Scripture

"Always be joyful. Never stop praying. Be thankful in all circumstances, for this is God's will for you who belong to Christ Jesus."
1 Thessalonians 5:16-18 NLT

Prayer

God, I come before you with a heart full of gratitude, recognizing the countless blessings you have poured into my life.

Affirmation

I will be grateful in whatever state I find myself.

Spiritual Growth
MILESTONES

-
-
-

Reflection

- "How does this verse speak to your current life situation?"

- "What does this verse reveal about God's character?"

- How does my daily life align with the word **GRATITUDE!**

Inspirational Quote

"Gratitude makes sense of our past, brings peace for today, and creates a vision for tomorrow".
~ Melody Beattie

My mental health
Monthly Check In

Date _____

Mo   Tu   We   Th   Fr   Sa   Su

What brings you Joy?

_____

_____

_____

How are you feeling this month?

😍 🙂 😐 🙁 😣

What did you worry about this month?

_____

_____

_____

Am I satisfied with this month?

😍 🙂 😐 🙁 😣

How are you taking care of yourself?

_____

_____

_____

Are you sleeping well?

😍 🙂 😐 🙁 😣

Habit Tracker

- ● Water
- ● Workout
- ● Take a walk
- ● Breathing exercises
- ● Meditation
- ● Read a book

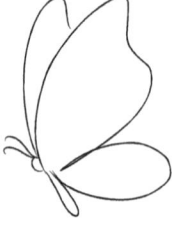

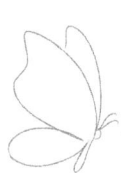

LORD MAKE ME OVER
TRANSFORMATIONAL *Journal*

Monthly Acronym

USING EACH LETTER, DESCRIBE A
TRANSFORMATIONAL EXPERIENCE

G _____

R _____

A _____

T _____

I _____

T _____

U _____

D _____

E _____

A Dose from Doc...

Gratitude

Living a life of gratitude to God opens your heart to His blessings and fills your soul with joy. Take time each day to thank Him—for His love, His faithfulness, and the little miracles around you. A grateful heart shines His light and reminds you of His goodness in every moment.

-Purpose Pusher-

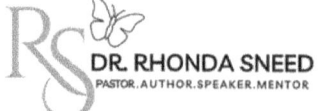

DR. RHONDA SNEED
PASTOR.AUTHOR.SPEAKER.MENTOR

INSPIRATIONAL AFFIRMATIONS

Gratitude

I choose to be thankful in all circumstances, knowing that God is with me in every season.
(1 Thessalonians 5:18)

I give thanks for all the blessings in my life, both big and small.

God's grace fills my heart with gratitude, and I will give thanks to Him daily. (Psalm 107:1)

I am grateful for God's presence, provision, and love in my life.

Today, I choose joy, peace, and positivity in all I do.

Choose or create affirmations that resonates deeply with you and reflects the mindset or attitude you wish to embody throughout your day. Repeat it to yourself as part of your morning routine, perhaps during meditation, while getting ready, or whenever it feels most effective for you. This repetition can help focus your mind and set a positive intention for the day ahead.

notes

_____

_____

_____

_____

_____

_____

_____

_____

_____

_____

notes

notes

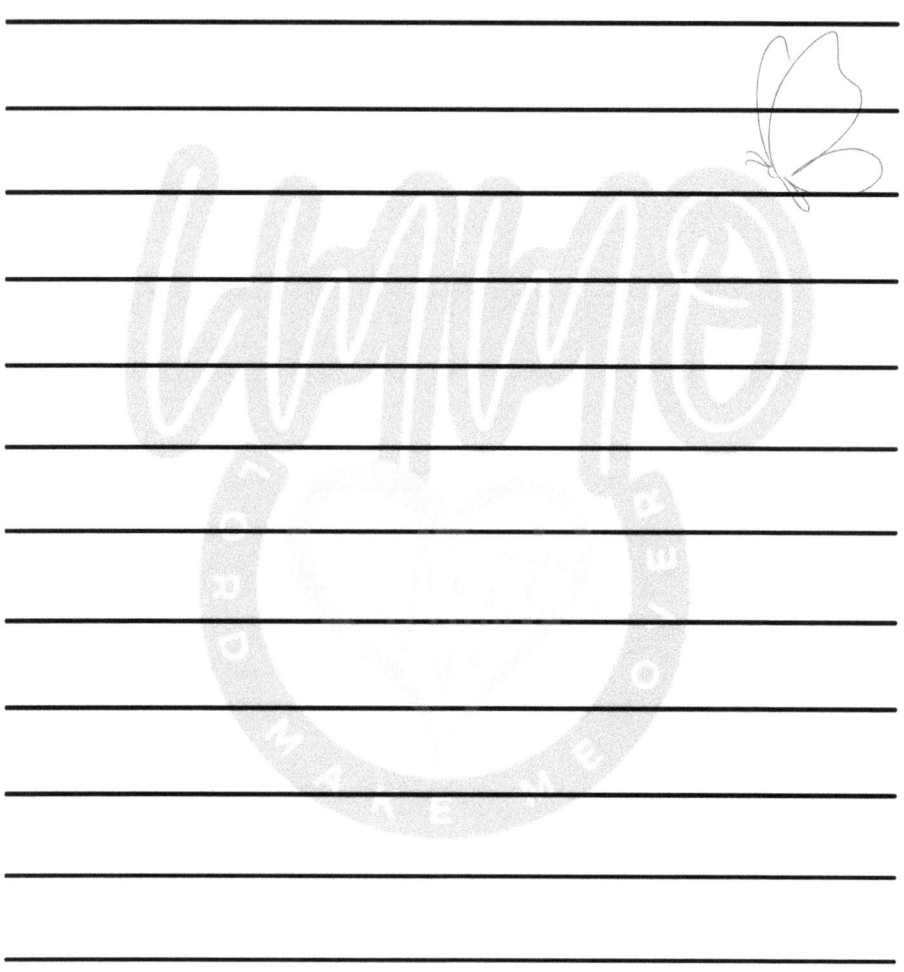

notes

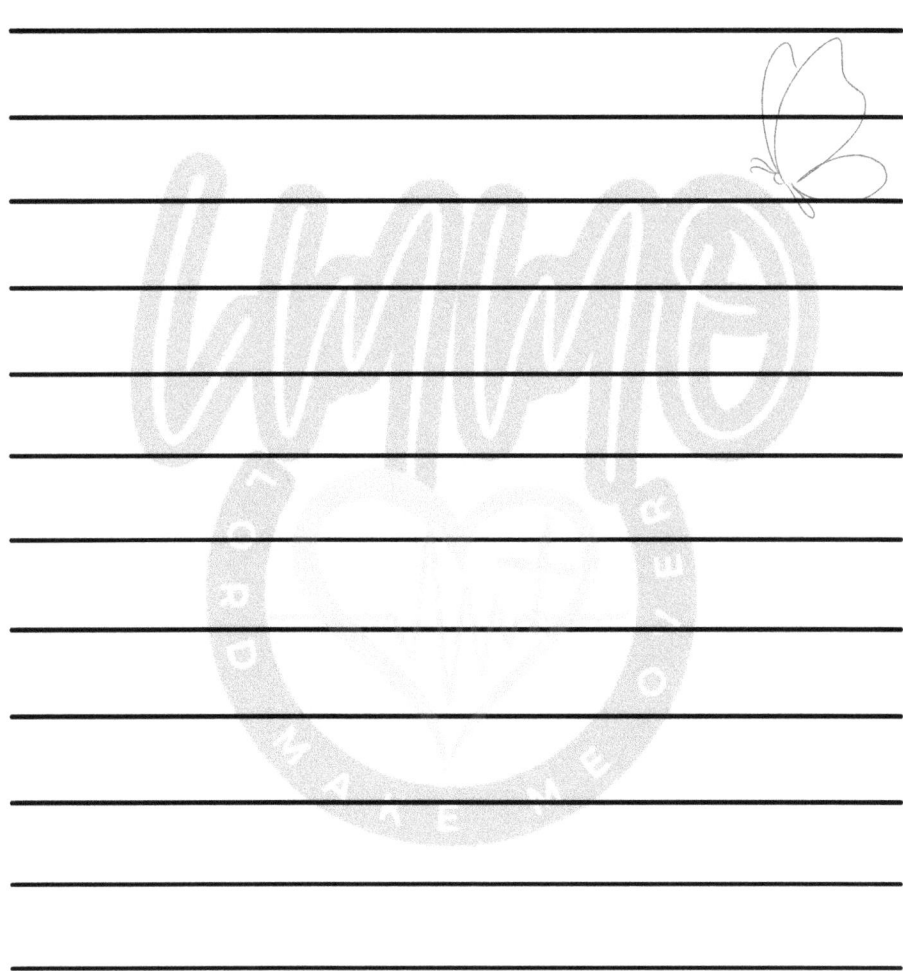

notes

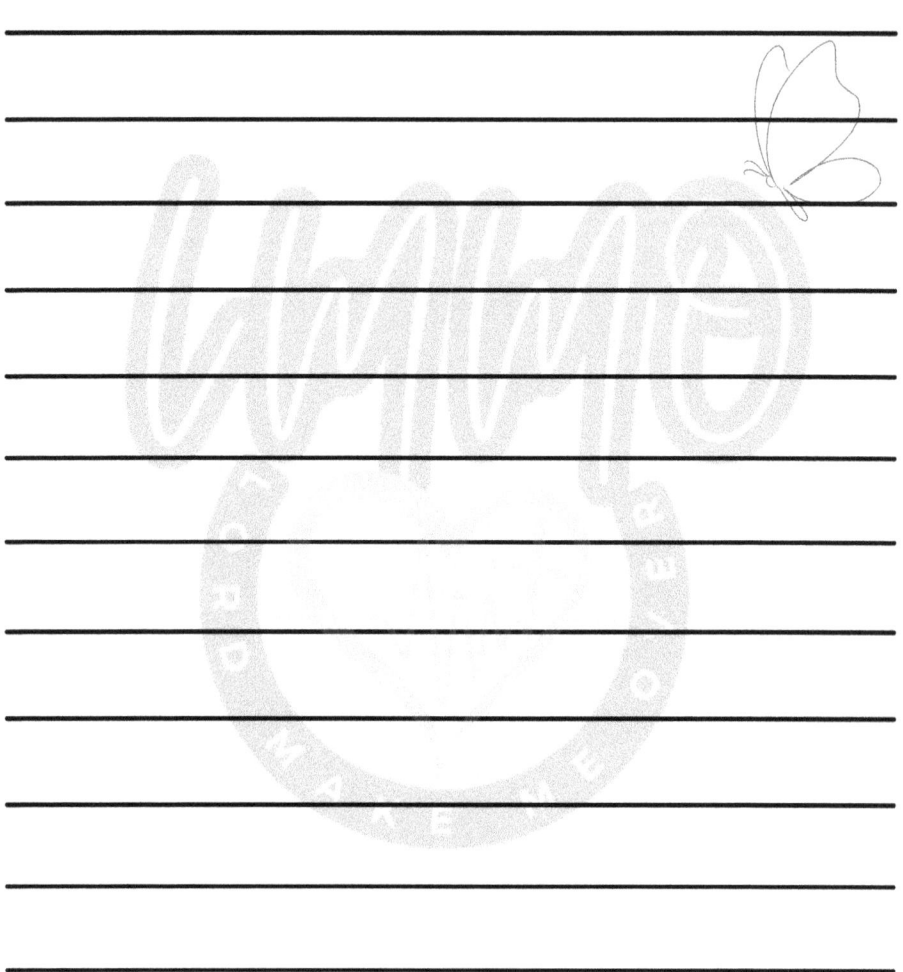

notes

_____

_____

_____

_____

_____

_____

_____

_____

_____

_____

Monthly
PLANNER

Month _____

OBEDIENCE

MON	TUE	WED	THU	FRI	SAT	SUN

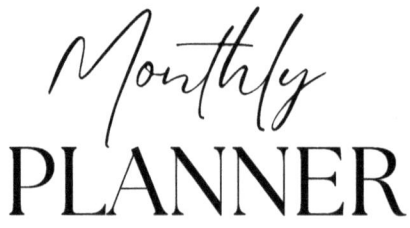

I'm grateful for: ---

Personal Testimonies:

Monthly Goal
◇ _____
◇ _____
◇ _____

OBEDIENCE

Scripture

"If you are willing and obedient, You shall eat the good of the land;"
Isaiah 1:19 NKJV

Prayer

God, I come before you today seeking a heart of true obedience, guide me to listen to your word and follow your commands with a willing spirit, help me to put your will first in all that I do."

Affirmation

I will obey God the first time.

Spiritual Growth
MILESTONES

-
-
-

Reflection

- "How does this verse speak to your current life situation?"

- "What does this verse reveal about God's character?"

- How does my daily life align with the word **OBEDIENCE**!

Inspirational Quote

"Obedience is the key to understanding God and it can open the way to God's revelations".
~ Oswald Chambers

My mental health
Monthly Check In

Date _____

Mo   Tu   We   Th   Fr   Sa   Su

What brings you Joy?

_____

_____

_____

How are you feeling this month?

😍 🙂 😐 😤 😣

_____

_____

What did you worry about this month?

_____

_____

_____

Am I satisfied with this month?

😍 🙂 😐 😤 😣

_____

_____

How are you taking care of yourself?

_____

_____

_____

Are you sleeping well?

😍 🙂 😐 😤 😣

_____

_____

Habit Tracker

- ● Water
- ● Workout
- ● Take a walk
- ● Breathing exercises
- ● Meditation
- ● Read a book

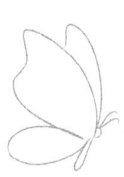

Monthly Acronym

USING EACH LETTER, DESCRIBE A
TRANSFORMATIONAL EXPERIENCE

O _____

B _____

E _____

D _____

I _____

E _____

N _____

C _____

E _____

A Dose from Doc...

Obedience

Living a life of obedience to God is a beautiful act of trust and love. His commands are not burdens but a guide to abundant living. When you follow His ways, you walk in His blessings and fulfill the purpose He's designed for you. Stay faithful, and He will honor your obedience in ways beyond what you can imagine.

-Purpose Pusher-

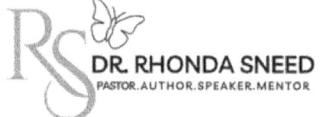

INSPIRATIONAL AFFIRMATIONS

Obedience

I choose to obey God, knowing that His commands are for my good and His glory. (John 14:15)

Obedience to God brings peace, joy, and fulfillment in my life.

I will follow God's direction, trusting that His way is always the best way.

I am obedient to God, knowing that He rewards those who follow His will. (Hebrews 11:6)

I will remain focused.

Choose or create affirmations that resonates deeply with you and reflects the mindset or attitude you wish to embody throughout your day. Repeat it to yourself as part of your morning routine, perhaps during meditation, while getting ready, or whenever it feels most effective for you. This repetition can help focus your mind and set a positive intention for the day ahead.

notes

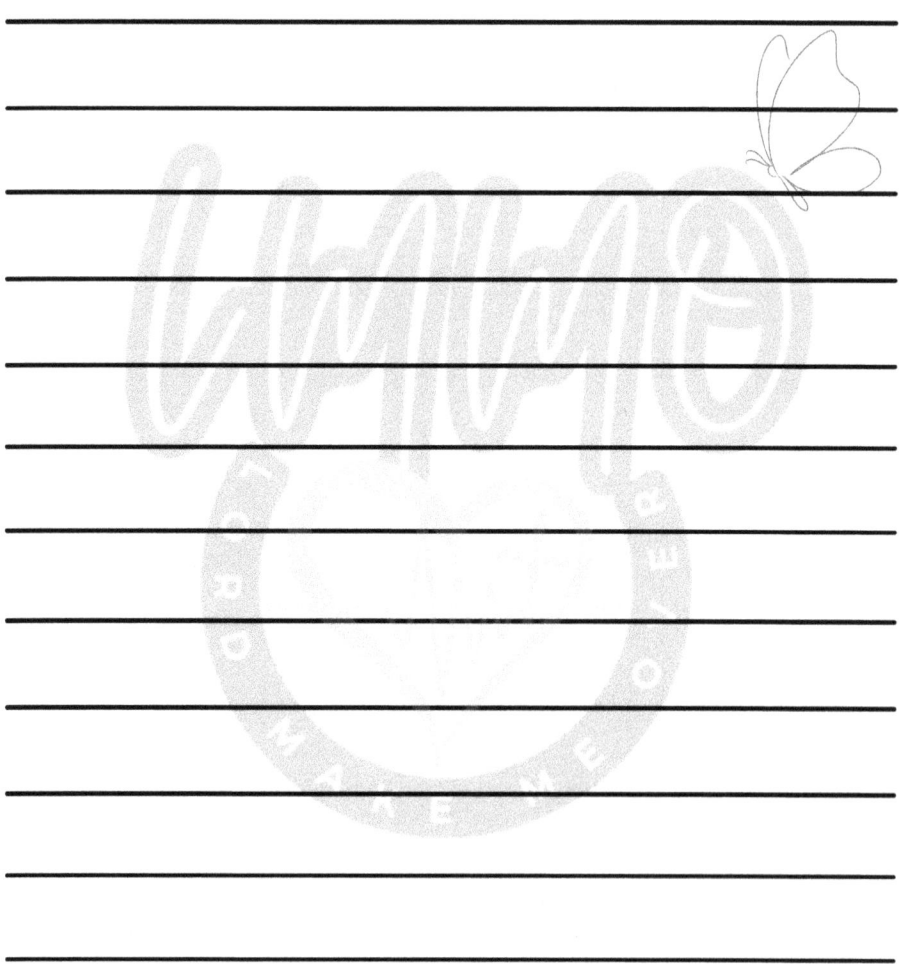

notes

LORD MAKE ME OVER
TRANSFORMATIONAL *Journal*

notes

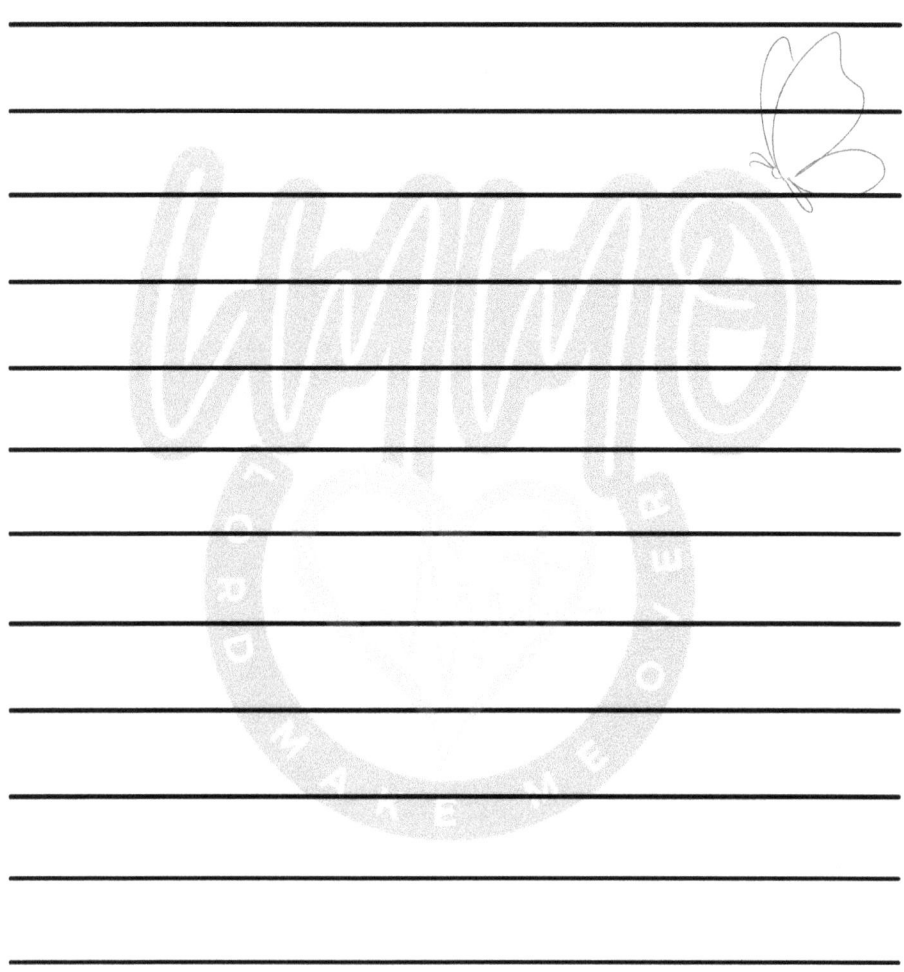

notes

notes

_____

_____

_____

_____

_____

_____

_____

_____

_____

_____

notes

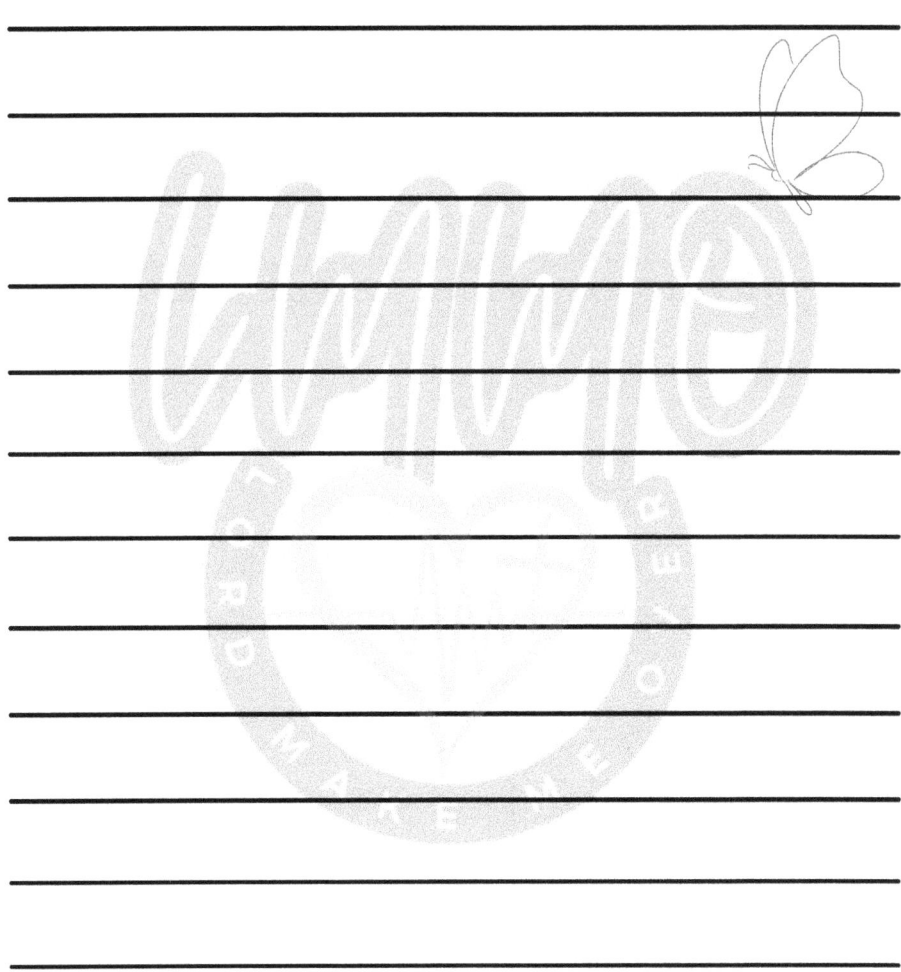

Monthly
PLANNER

Month _____

WISDOM

MON	TUE	WED	THU	FRI	SAT	SUN

I'm grateful for: --

Personal Testimonies:

Monthly Goal

◇ _____

◇ _____

◇ _____

WISDOM

Scripture

"Get all the advice and instructions you can, so you will be wise the rest of your life."
Proverbs 19:20 NLT

Prayer

God, I humbly ask that You grant me wisdom and a discerning spirit to make sound choices and decisions.

Affirmation

I will make wise decisions.

Spiritual Growth
MILESTONES

-
-
-

Reflection

- "How does this verse speak to your current life situation?"

- "What does this verse reveal about God's character?"

- How does my daily life align with the word **WISDOM**!

Inspirational Quote

"Wisdom is not a product of schooling but of the lifelong attempt to acquire it."
~ Albert Einstein

My mental health
Monthly Check In

Date _____

Mo   Tu   We   Th   Fr   Sa   Su

What brings you Joy?

_____

_____

_____

How are you feeling this month?

😍 😊 😐 😟 😖

_____

_____

What did you worry about this month?

_____

_____

_____

Am I satisfied with this month?

😍 😊 😐 😟 😖

_____

_____

How are you taking care of yourself?

_____

_____

_____

Are you sleeping well?

😍 😊 😐 😟 😖

_____

_____

Habit Tracker

- ⚫ Water
- ⚫ Workout
- ⚫ Take a walk
- ⚫ Breathing exercises
- ⚫ Meditation
- ⚫ Read a book

A Dose from Doc...

Wisdom

When you ask God for wisdom, you're inviting His guidance into your life. He promises to give it generously to those who seek it. Trust Him to provide clarity, insight, and direction for every decision. Lean on His wisdom, and He will lead you on the right path.

-Purpose Pusher-

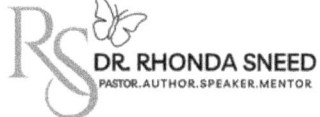

DR. RHONDA SNEED
PASTOR.AUTHOR.SPEAKER.MENTOR

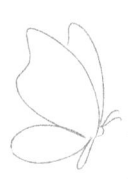

Monthly Acronym

USING EACH LETTER, DESCRIBE A
TRANSFORMATIONAL EXPERIENCE

W _____

I _____

S _____

D _____

O _____

M _____

INSPIRATIONAL
AFFIRMATIONS
Wisdom

I seek God's wisdom in every decision, trusting that He will guide me with understanding. (James 1:5)

God's wisdom is more precious than silver or gold, and I will seek it daily. (Proverbs 3:13-15)

I trust that God's wisdom will illuminate my path and lead me to success.

I will walk in God's wisdom, knowing it brings life and peace.

I am in control of my thoughts, emotions, and actions today.

Choose or create affirmations that resonates deeply with you and reflects the mindset or attitude you wish to embody throughout your day. Repeat it to yourself as part of your morning routine, perhaps during meditation, while getting ready, or whenever it feels most effective for you. This repetition can help focus your mind and set a positive intention for the day ahead.

notes

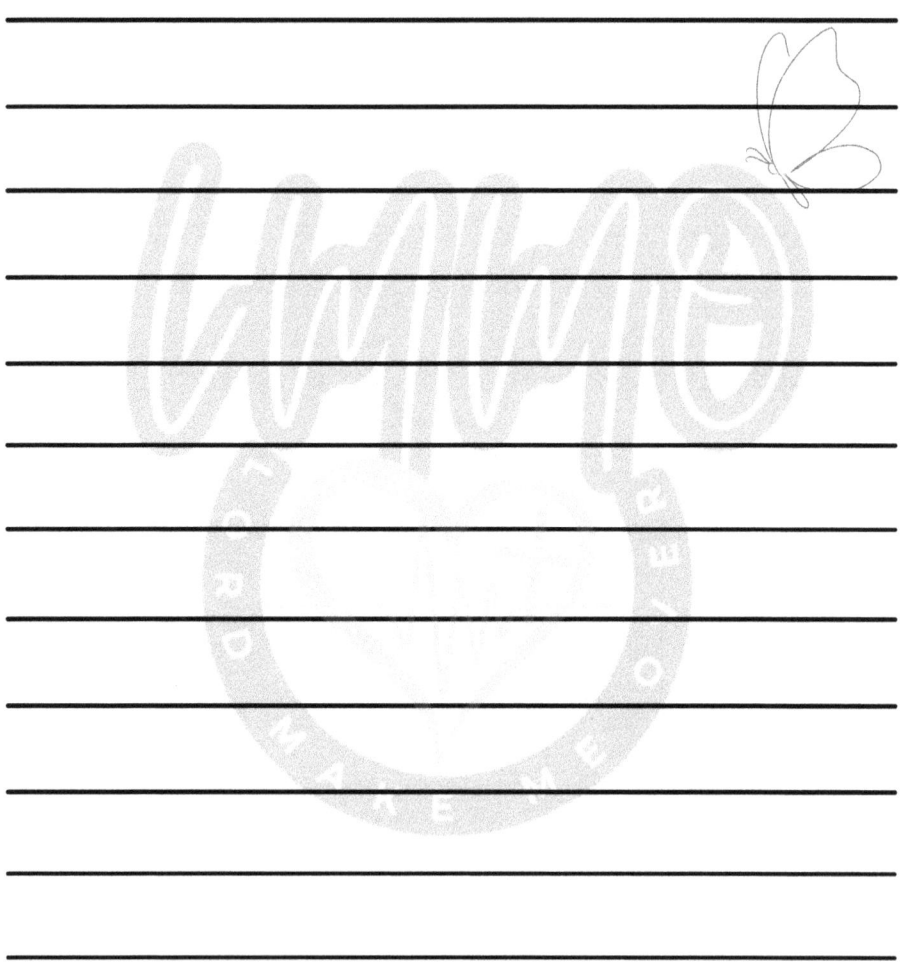

_____

_____

_____

_____

_____

_____

_____

_____

_____

_____

notes

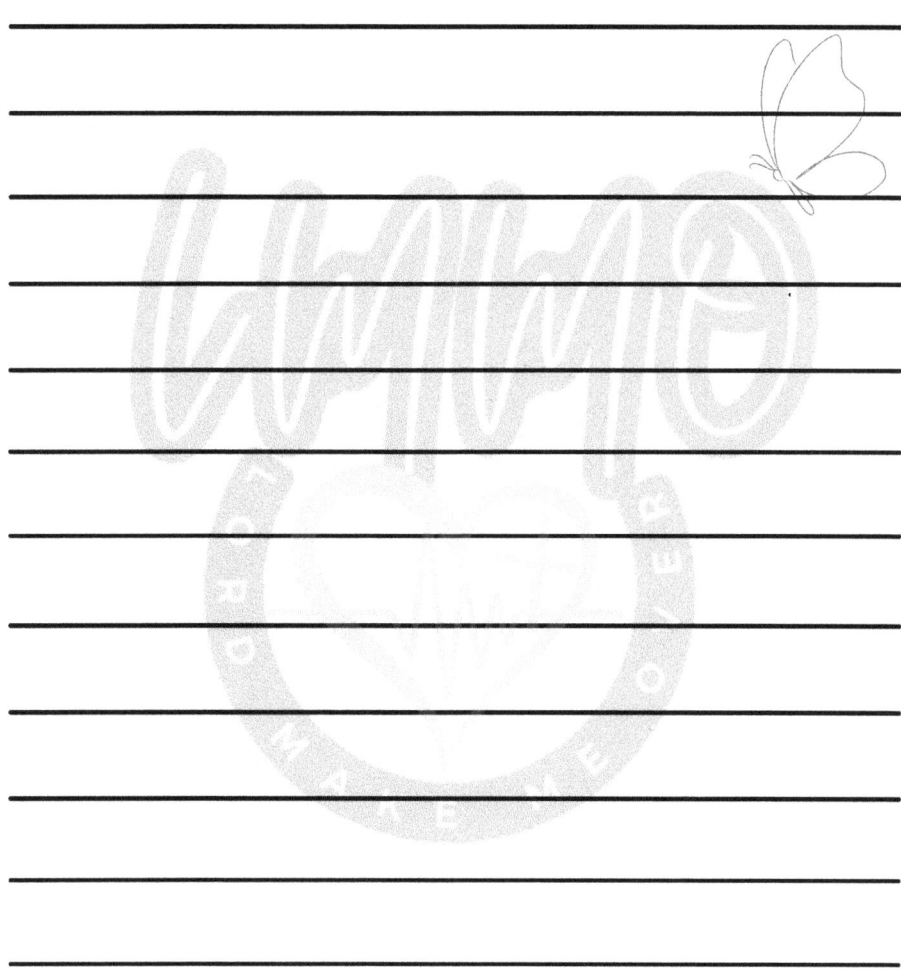

notes

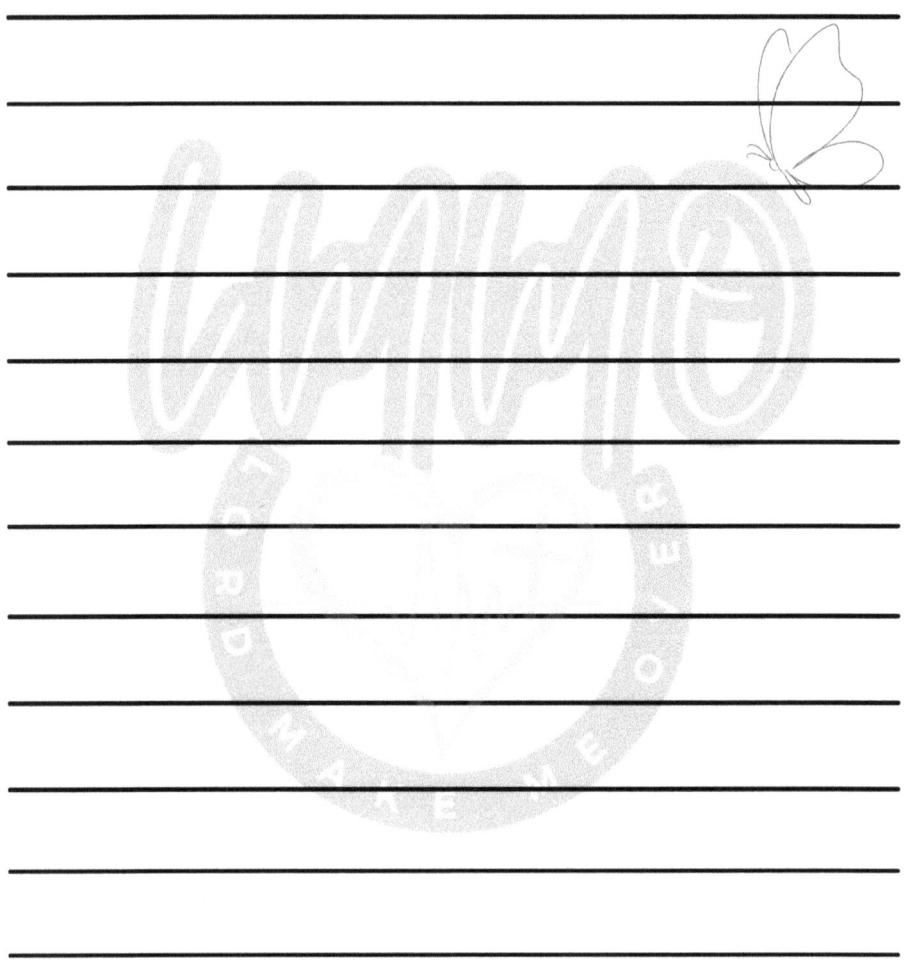

_____

_____

_____

_____

_____

_____

_____

_____

_____

_____

notes

notes

_____

_____

_____

_____

_____

_____

_____

_____

_____

_____

notes

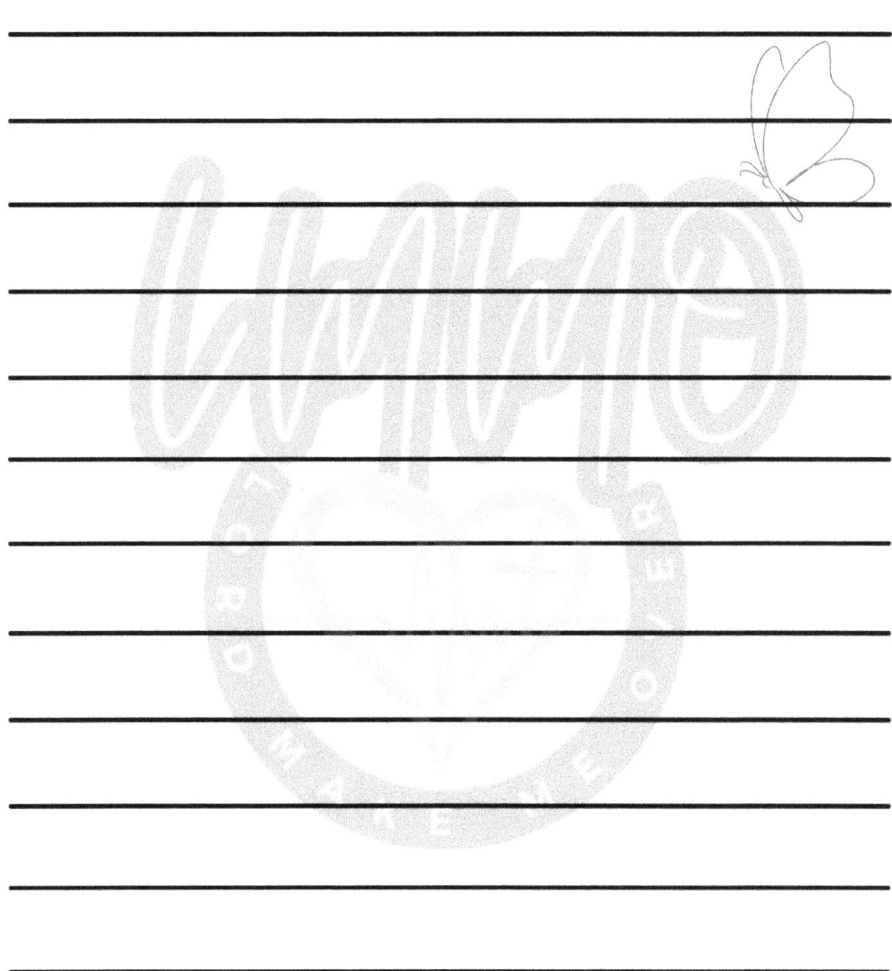

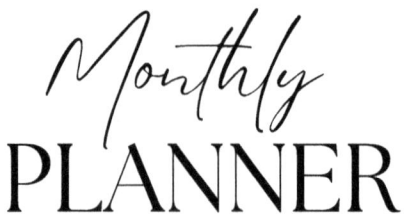

Monthly
PLANNER

Month _____

SURRENDER

MON	TUE	WED	THU	FRI	SAT	SUN

I'm grateful for: ---

Personal Testimonies:

Monthly Goal
_____
◇ _____
◇ _____
◇ _____

SURRENDER

Scripture

"Therefore humble yourselves under the mighty hand of God, that He may exalt you in due time, casting all your care upon Him, for He cares for you."
I Peter 5:6-7 NKJV

Prayer

Lord, I surrender my whole life to you, the past, the present, and the future. In sickness and in health, in life and in death, I belong to you.

Affirmation

I surrender all of me to you, God.

Spiritual Growth MILESTONES

-
-
-

Reflection

- "How does this verse speak to your current life situation?"

- "What does this verse reveal about God's character?"

- How does my daily life align with the word **SURRENDER**!

Inspirational Quote

"The moment of surrender is not when life is over, it's when it begins." ~ Marianne Williamson

My mental health
Monthly Check In

Date _____

Mo   Tu   We   Th   Fr   Sa   Su

What brings you Joy?

_____

_____

_____

How are you feeling this month?

_____

_____

What did you worry about this month?

_____

_____

_____

Am I satisfied with this month?

😍 😊 😐 🙁 😞

_____

_____

How are you taking care of yourself?

_____

_____

_____

Are you sleeping well?

😍 😊 😐 🙁 😞

_____

_____

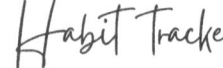

Habit Tracker

- ● Water
- ● Workout
- ● Take a walk
- ● Breathing exercises
- ● Meditation
- ● Read a book

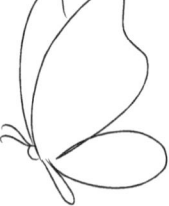

A Dose from Doc...

Surrender

Surrendering to God is not a sign of weakness but an act of trust and strength. When you let go of control and give everything to Him, you make room for His peace, guidance, and blessings to fill your life. Trust that His plans are greater, and He will lead you in love and purpose.

-Purpose Pusher-

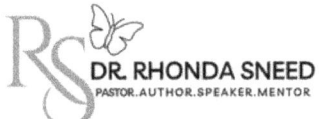

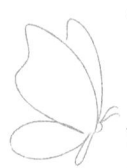

Monthly Acronym

USING EACH LETTER, DESCRIBE A
TRANSFORMATIONAL EXPERIENCE

S _____

U _____

R _____

R _____

E _____

N _____

D _____

E _____

R _____

INSPIRATIONAL AFFIRMATIONS

Surrender

I surrender my plans to God, trusting that His will is always best for me. (Matthew 16:24)

I surrender my worries, knowing that God is in control and will take care of me.

In surrender, I find peace, because I trust that God is faithful to provide.

I choose to let go and allow God to lead me in His perfect way.

Today will be a productive day.

Choose or create affirmations that resonates deeply with you and reflects the mindset or attitude you wish to embody throughout your day. Repeat it to yourself as part of your morning routine, perhaps during meditation, while getting ready, or whenever it feels most effective for you. This repetition can help focus your mind and set a positive intention for the day ahead.

notes

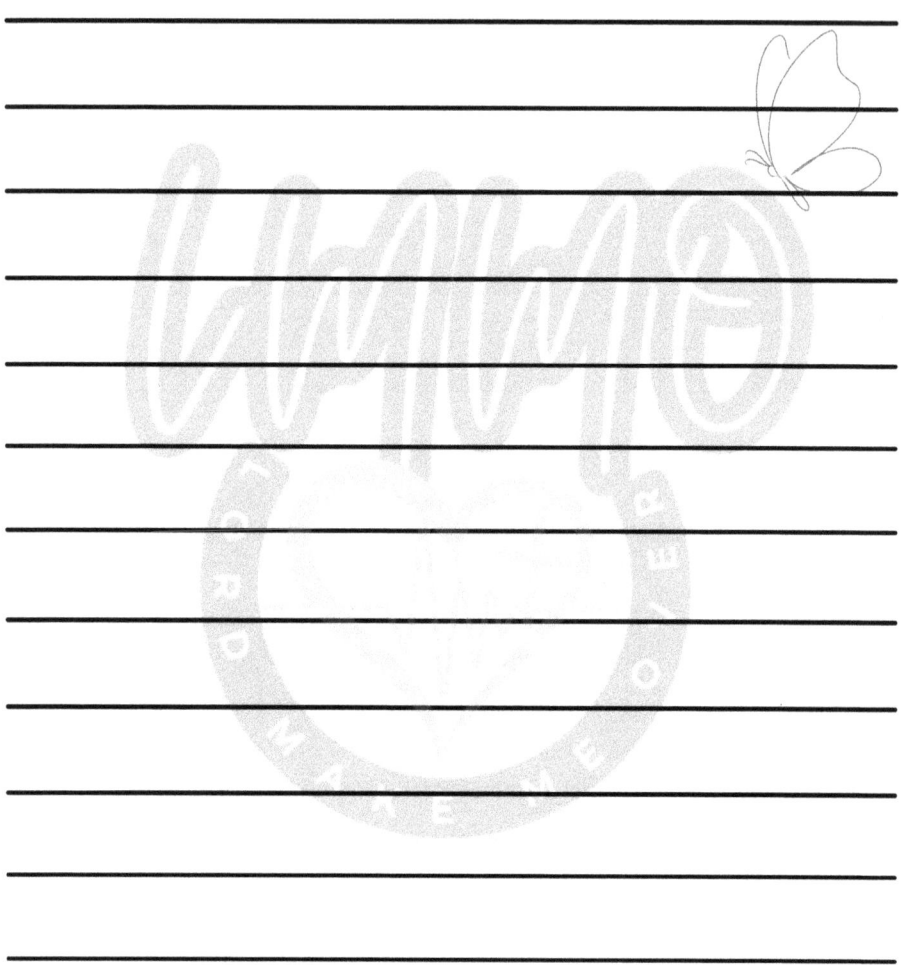

notes

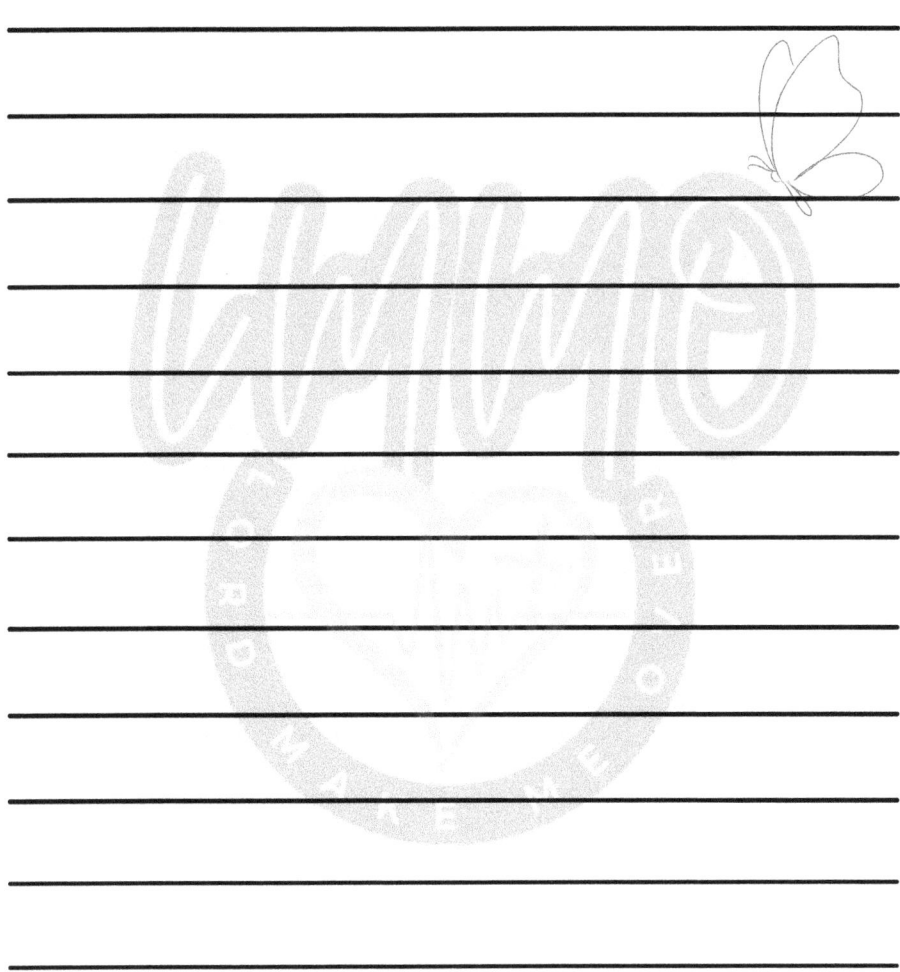

notes

notes

notes

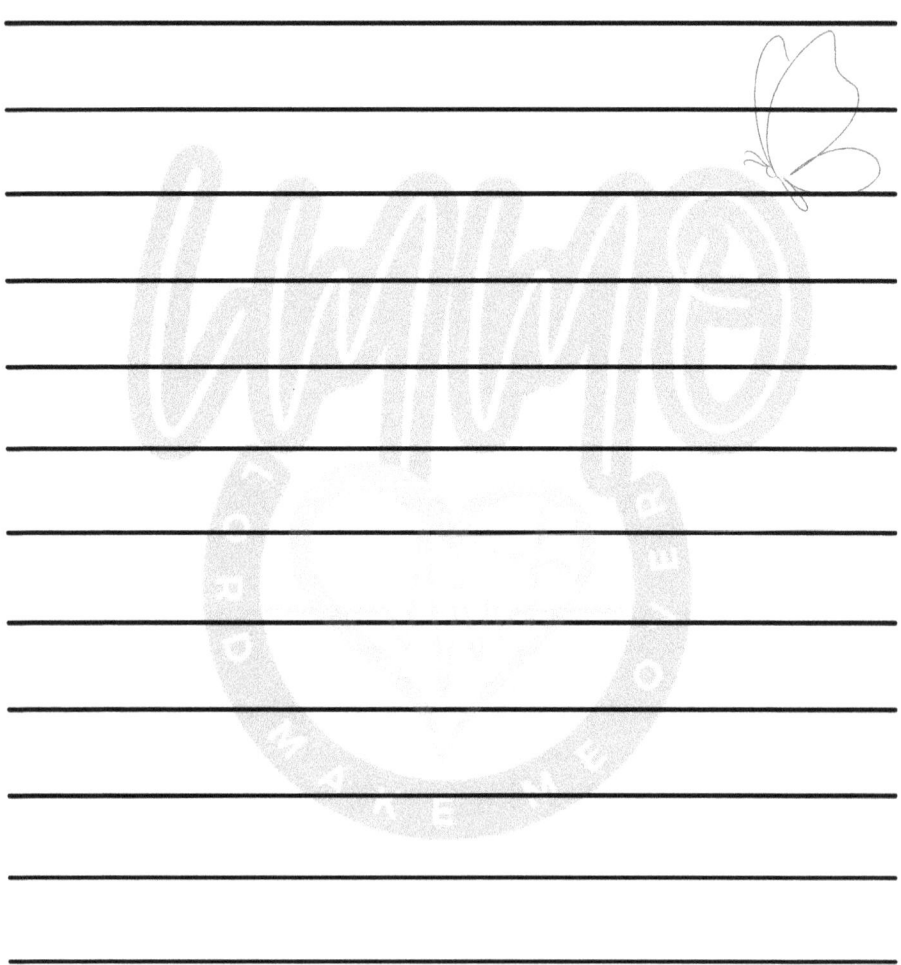

_____

_____

_____

_____

_____

_____

_____

_____

_____

_____

notes

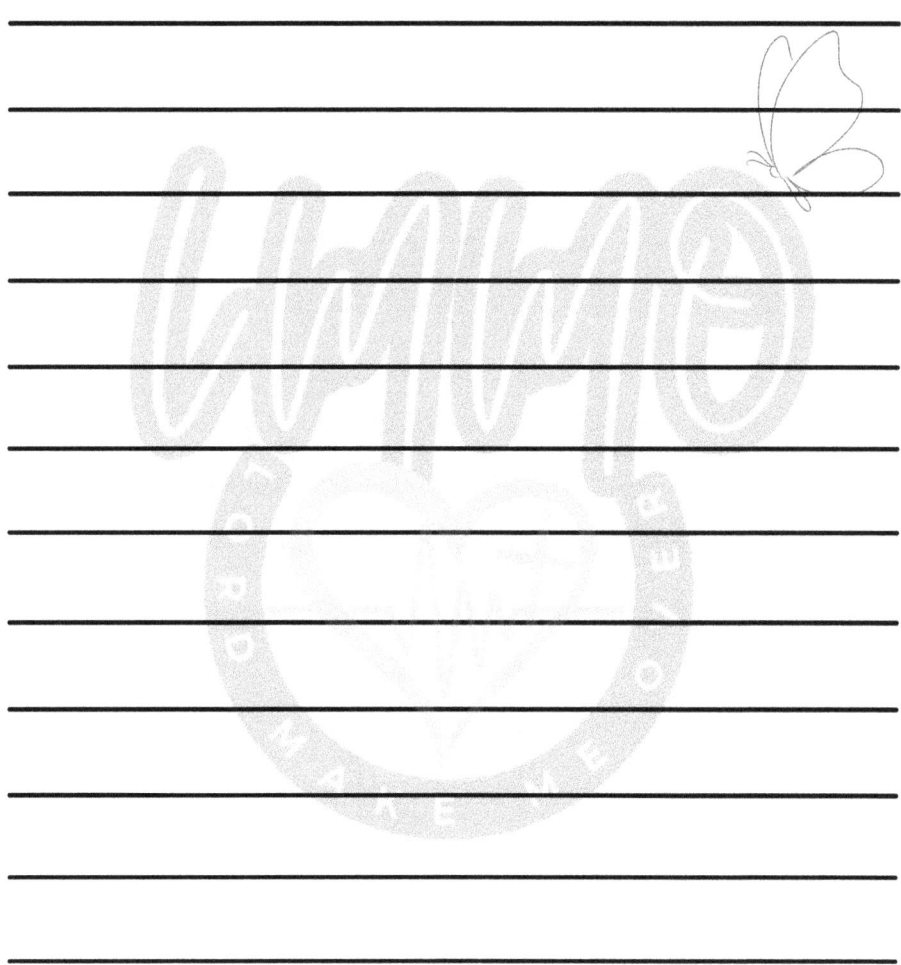

_____

_____

_____

_____

_____

_____

_____

_____

_____

_____

_____

Monthly
PLANNER

Month _____

PEACE

MON	TUE	WED	THU	FRI	SAT	SUN

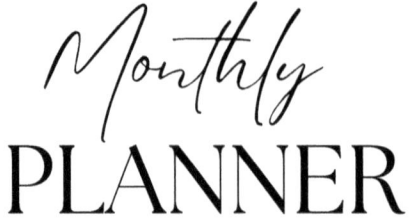

I'm grateful for: --

Personal Testimonies:

Monthly Goal

◇ _____

◇ _____

◇ _____

PEACE

Scripture

"You will keep in perfect peace all who trust in you, all whose thoughts are fixed on you!"
Isaiah 26:3 NLT

Prayer

God, I ask you to give me peace in my mind, body, soul and spirit. I need you to heal and remove everything that is causing stress, grief, and sorrow in my life.

Affirmation

I will protect my peace.

Spiritual Growth
MILESTONES

-
-
-

Reflection

- "How does this verse speak to your current life situation?"

- "What does this verse reveal about God's character?"

- How does my daily life align with the word **PEACE**!

Inspirational Quote

"If you cannot find peace within yourself, you will never find it anywhere else." ~ Marvin Gaye

My mental health
Monthly Check In

Date _____

Mo   Tu   We   Th   Fr   Sa   Su

What brings you Joy?

_____

_____

_____

How are you feeling this month?

😍 😊 😐 😣 😖

_____

_____

What did you worry about this month?

_____

_____

_____

Am I satisfied with this month?

😍 😊 😐 😣 😖

_____

_____

How are you taking care of yourself?

_____

_____

_____

Are you sleeping well?

😍 😊 😐 😣 😖

_____

_____

Habit Tracker

● Water
● Workout
● Take a walk
● Breathing exercises
● Meditation
● Read a book

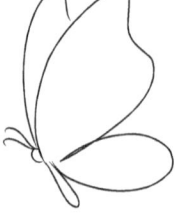

A Dose from Doc...

Peace

Walking in the peace of God begins with trusting Him fully. Let go of worry and choose to rest in His presence, knowing He holds every moment of your life in His hands. His peace surpasses all understanding, guarding your heart and mind. Stay close to Him, and His peace will guide you through every situation. Make a choice to protect your peace.

-Purpose Pusher-

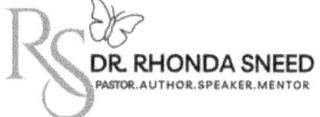

DR. RHONDA SNEED
PASTOR.AUTHOR.SPEAKER.MENTOR

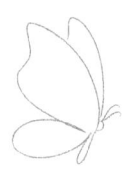

Monthly Acronym

USING EACH LETTER, DESCRIBE A
TRANSFORMATIONAL EXPERIENCE

P _____

E _____

A _____

C _____

E _____

INSPIRATIONAL AFFIRMATIONS

Peace

I receive the peace of God, which surpasses all understanding, to guard my heart and mind. (Philippians 4:7)

In Christ, I have peace, and I will not let fear or anxiety control me. (John 14:27)

God's peace fills my heart and guides my thoughts, leading me to rest in Him.

I walk in peace, knowing that God is my refuge and strength.

I will protect my peace.

Choose or create affirmations that resonates deeply with you and reflects the mindset or attitude you wish to embody throughout your day. Repeat it to yourself as part of your morning routine, perhaps during meditation, while getting ready, or whenever it feels most effective for you. This repetition can help focus your mind and set a positive intention for the day ahead.

notes

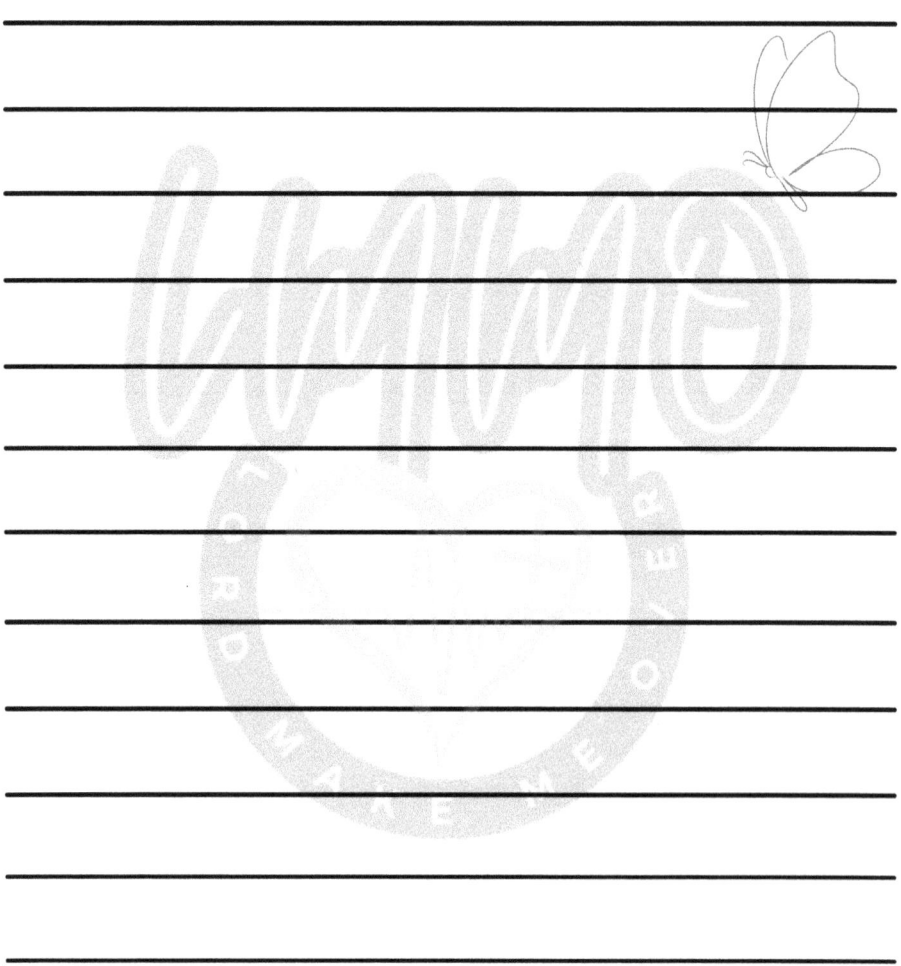

---

notes

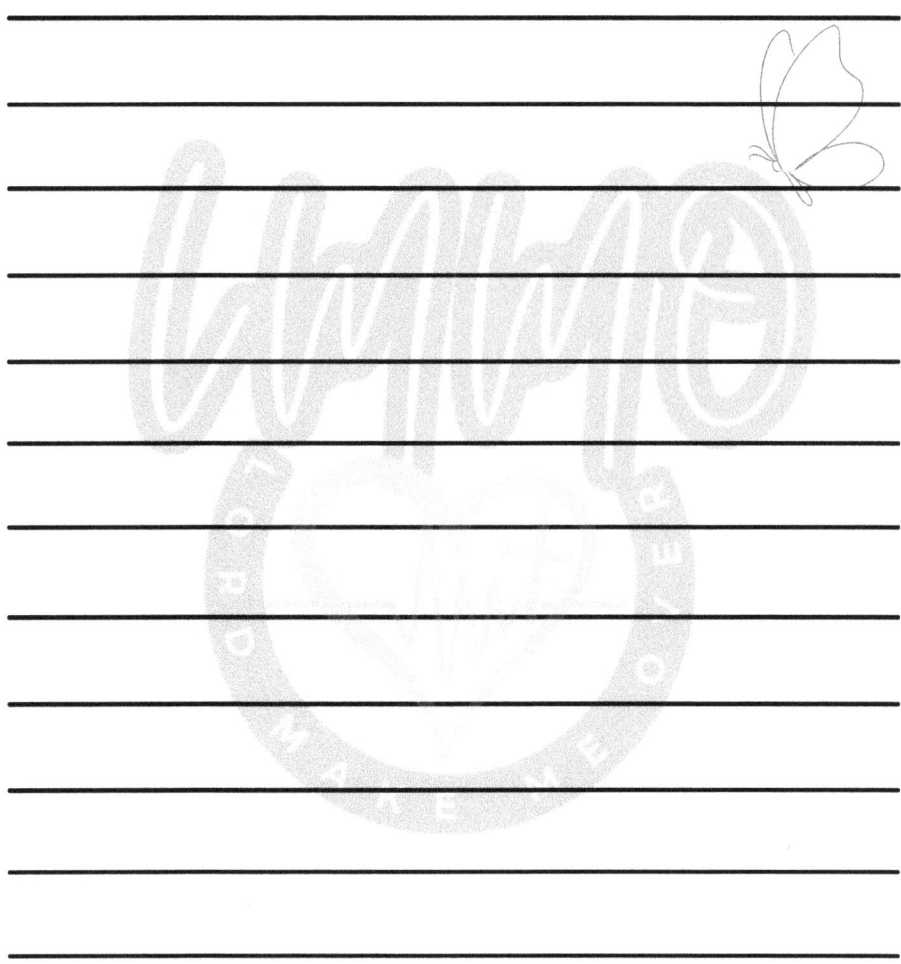

_____

_____

_____

_____

_____

_____

_____

_____

_____

_____

_____

notes

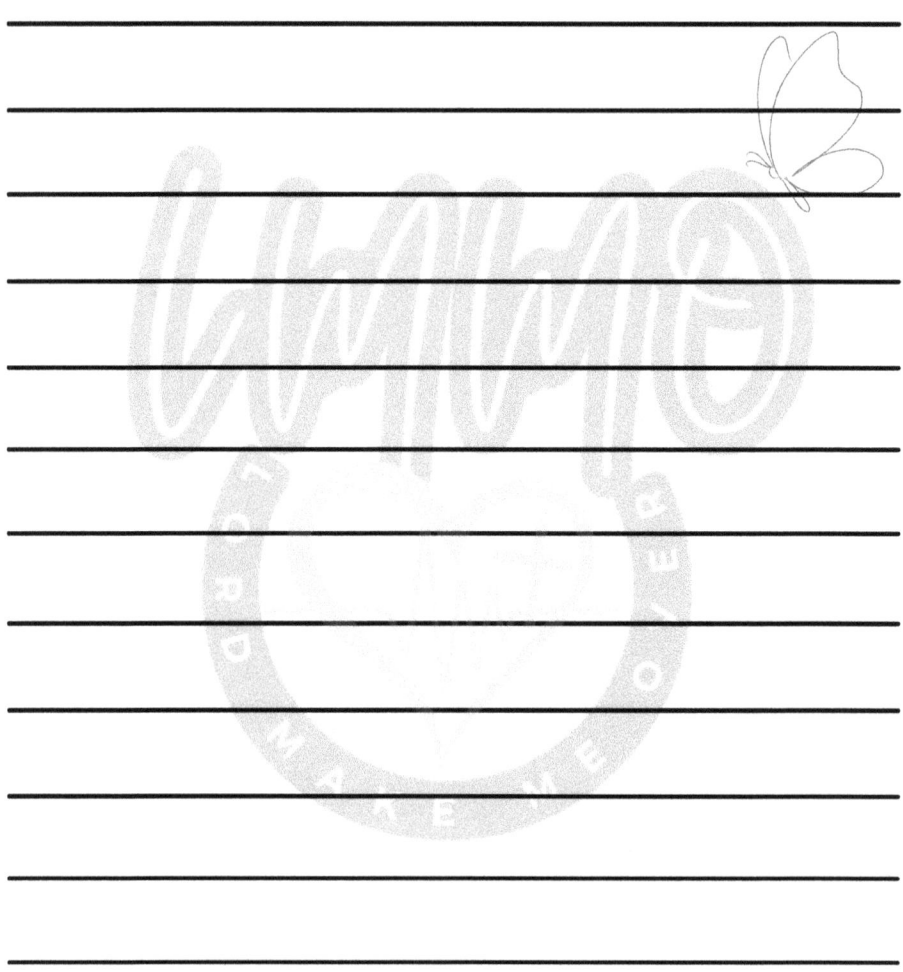

notes

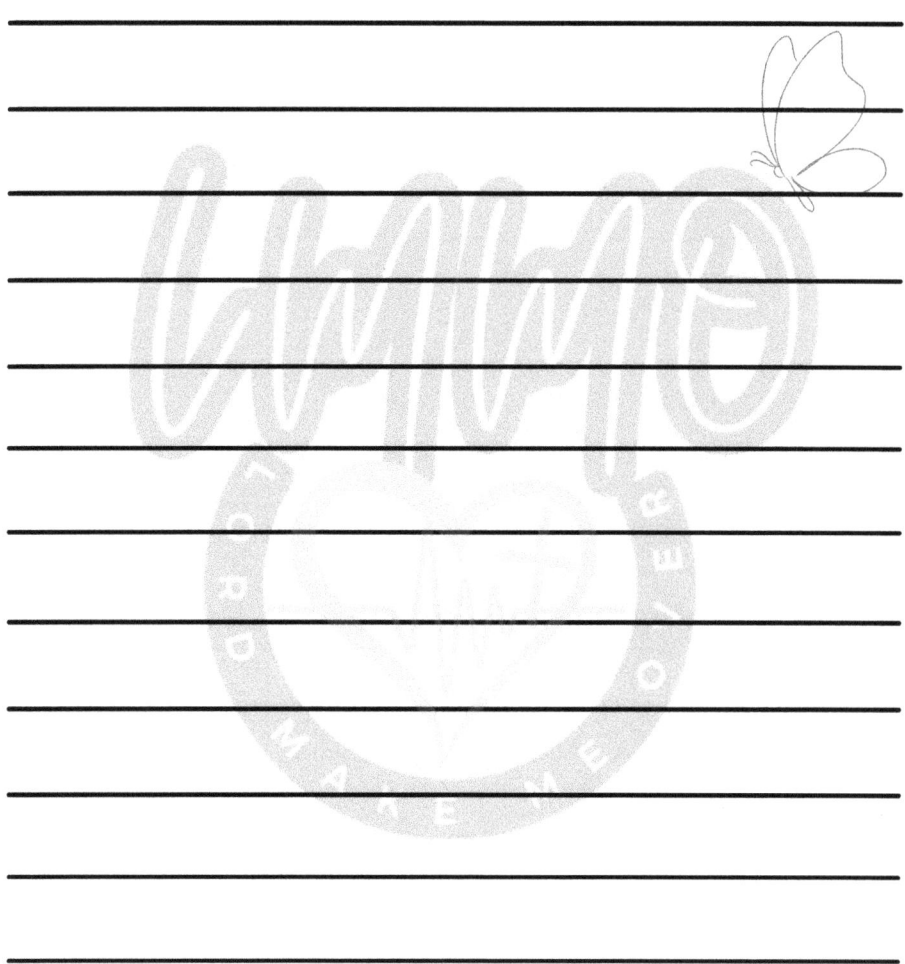

_____

_____

_____

_____

_____

_____

_____

_____

_____

_____

_____

notes

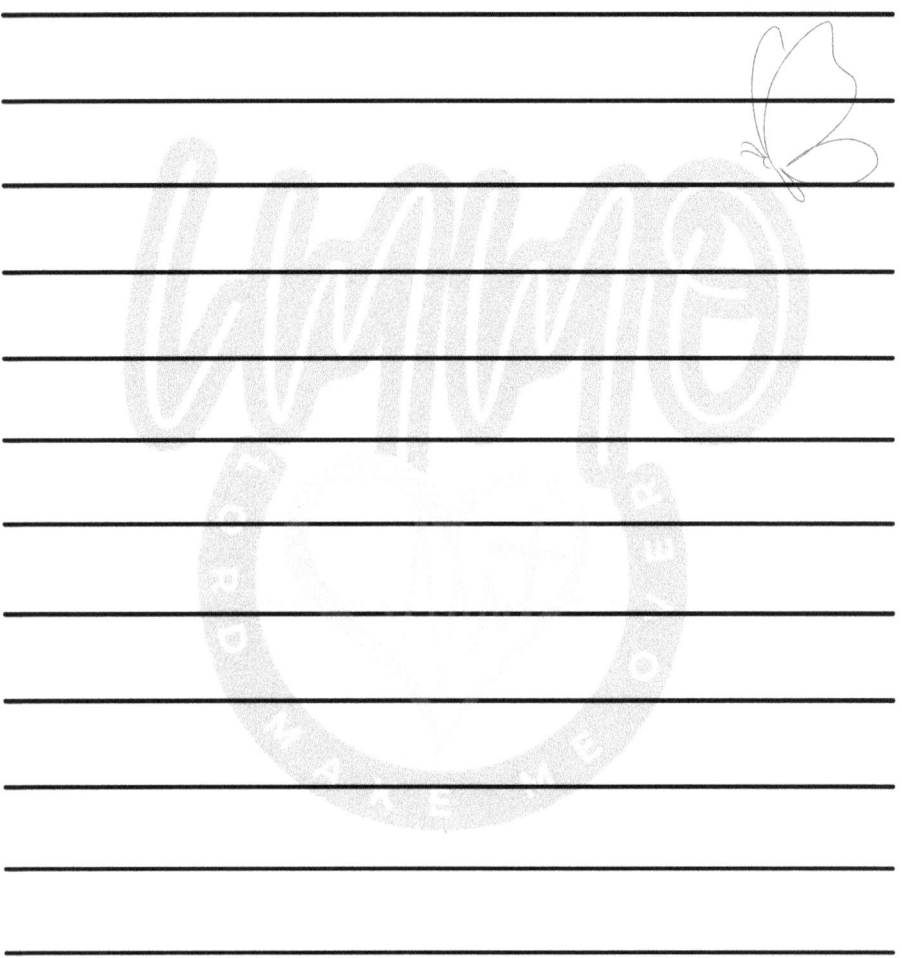

_____

_____

_____

_____

_____

_____

_____

_____

_____

_____

notes

Monthly PLANNER

Month _____

GRACE

MON	TUE	WED	THU	FRI	SAT	SUN

I'm grateful for: _____

_____

Personal Testimonies:

Monthly Goal

◇ _____

◇ _____

◇ _____

GRACE

Scripture

"But whatever I am now, it is all because God poured out his special favor on me—and not without results. For I have worked harder than any of the other apostles; yet it was not I but God who was working through me by his grace."
1 Corinthians 15:10 NLT

Prayer

God, I bless you for my life, I give you praise for your abundant mercy and grace towards me. I thank you for your faithfulness even though I am not always faithful to you. Thank you for paying the ultimate sacrifice that I may come into relationship with you. Help me to live in your victory over sin and death.

Affirmation

I will extend grace to others just as God does for me.

Spiritual Growth MILESTONES

- •
- •
- •

Reflection

- "How does this verse speak to your current life situation?"

- "What does this verse reveal about God's character?"

- How does my daily life align with the word **GRACE**!

Inspirational Quote

"**GRACE means that all of your mistakes now serve a purpose instead of serving shame**".
~ Brené Brown

My mental health
Monthly Check In

Date _____

Mo   Tu   We   Th   Fr   Sa   Su

What brings you Joy?

_____

_____

_____

How are you feeling this month?

😍 🙂 😐 😖 😧

_____

_____

What did you worry about this month?

_____

_____

_____

Am I satisfied with this month?

😍 🙂 😐 😖 😧

_____

_____

How are you taking care of yourself?

_____

_____

_____

Are you sleeping well?

😍 🙂 😐 😖 😧

_____

_____

Habit Tracker

- ⬤ Water
- ⬤ Workout
- ⬤ Take a walk
- ⬤ Breathing exercises
- ⬤ Meditation
- ⬤ Read a book

A Dose from Doc...

Grace

Show the grace of God by extending kindness, forgiveness, and compassion to others, just as He has shown you. When you reflect His grace, you become a living example of His love and mercy. Remember, grace is not earned, but given—freely share it, and watch how it transforms lives, starting with your own.

-Purpose Pusher-

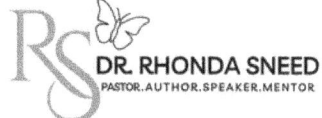

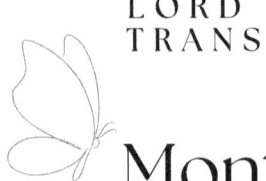

Monthly Acronym

USING EACH LETTER, DESCRIBE A TRANSFORMATIONAL EXPERIENCE

G _____

R _____

A _____

C _____

E _____

INSPIRATIONAL AFFIRMATIONS

Grace

God's grace is sufficient for me in every moment, and His power is made perfect in my weakness."
(2 Corinthians 12:9)

I receive God's grace with a humble heart, knowing I am unworthy but loved beyond measure.

God's grace transforms me, empowers me, and equips me for the life He has called me to live.

I am saved by grace through faith, and I am eternally grateful for God's unmerited favor. (Ephesians 2:8-9)

I am capable of achieving my goals.

Choose or create affirmations that resonates deeply with you and reflects the mindset or attitude you wish to embody throughout your day. Repeat it to yourself as part of your morning routine, perhaps during meditation, while getting ready, or whenever it feels most effective for you. This repetition can help focus your mind and set a positive intention for the day ahead.

notes

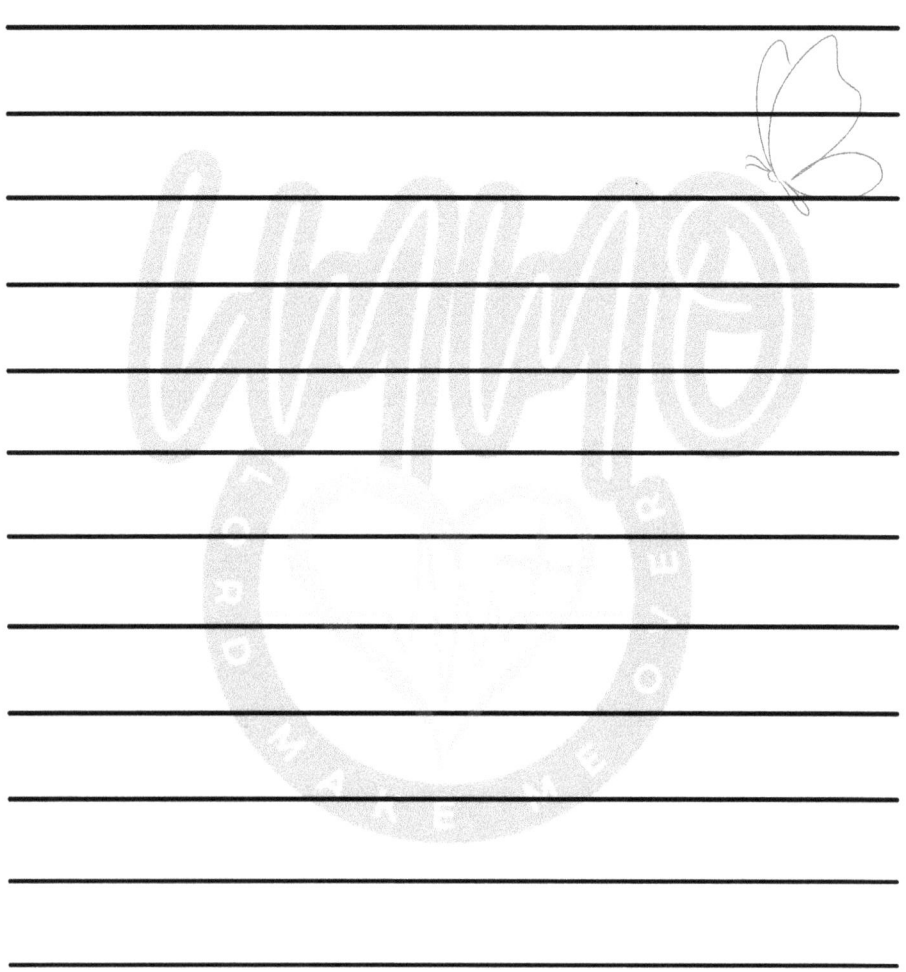

notes

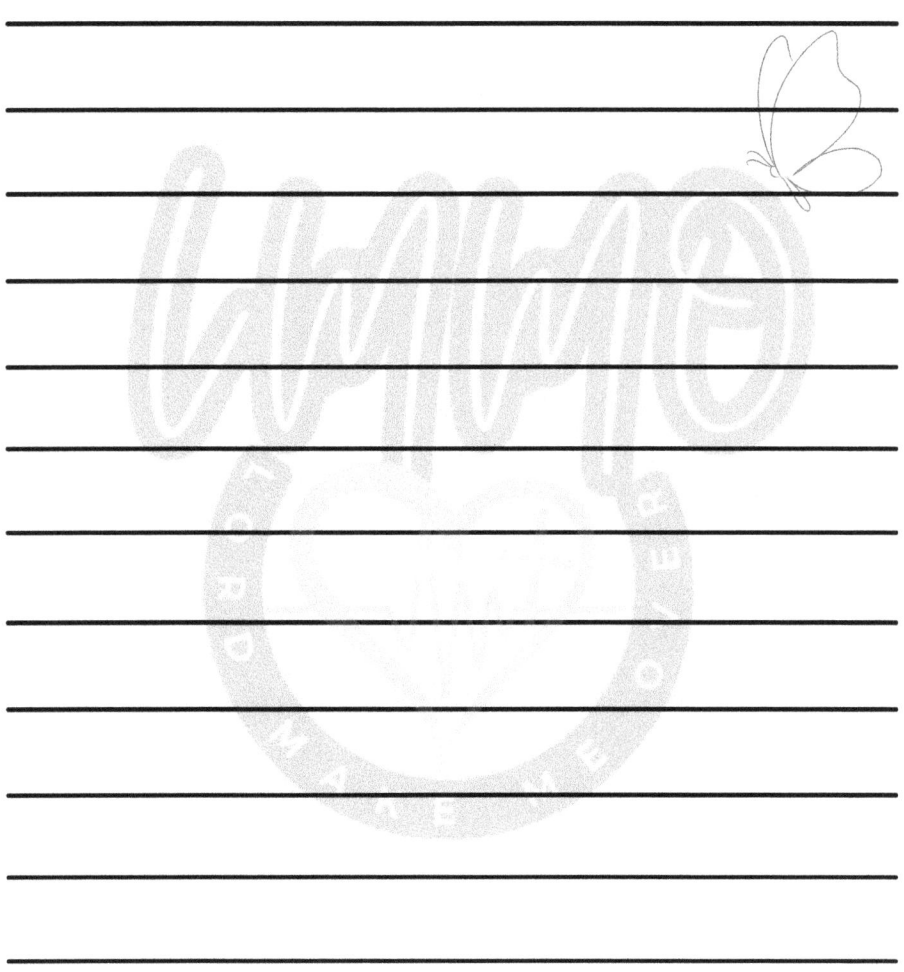

notes

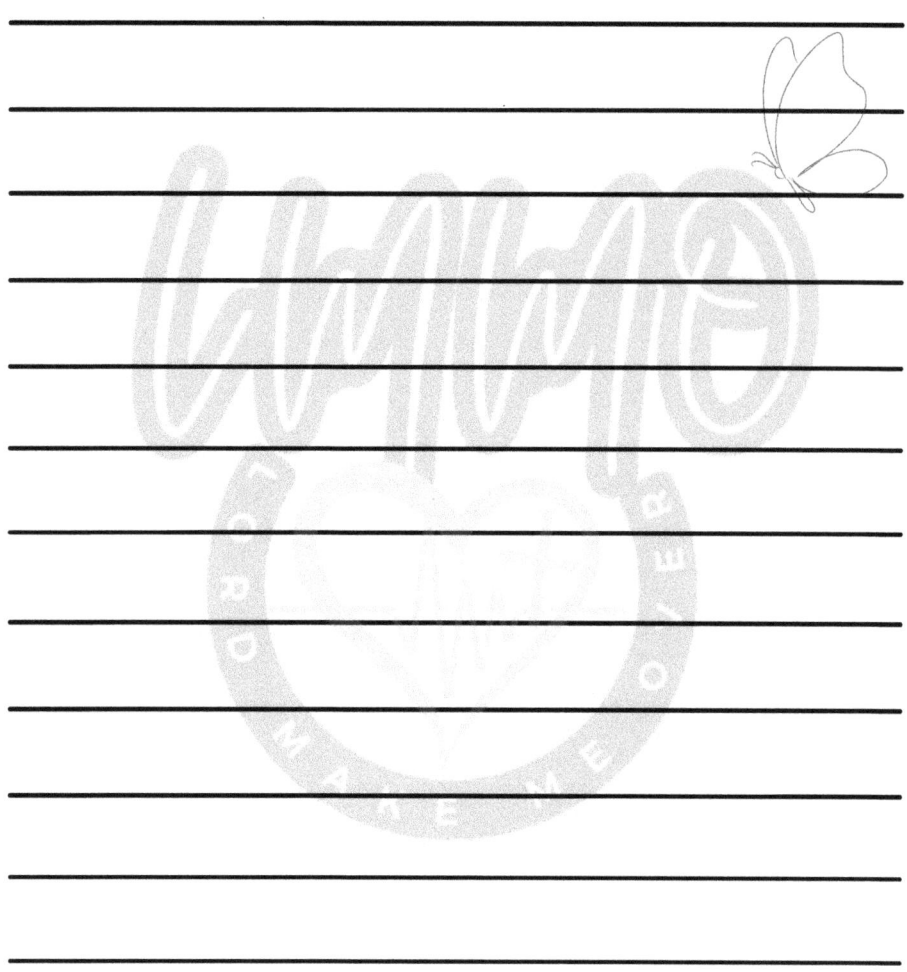

notes

_____

_____

_____

_____

_____

_____

_____

_____

_____

_____

_____

notes

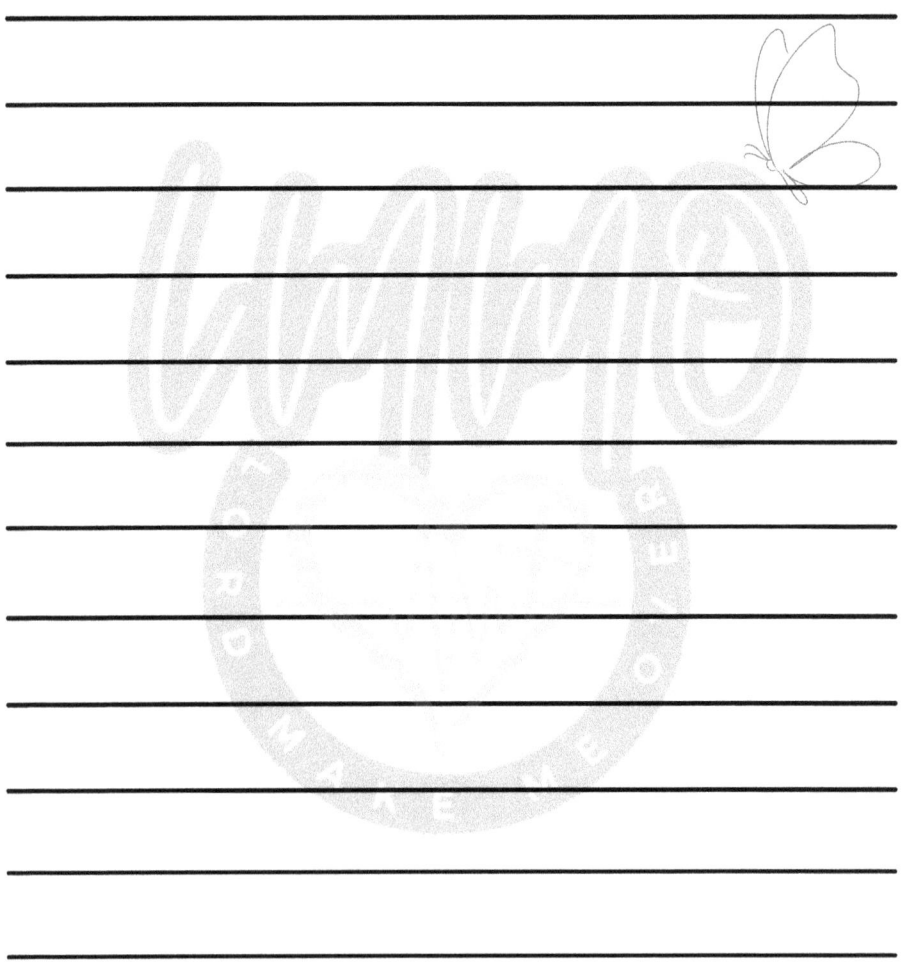

LORD MAKE ME OVER
TRANSFORMATIONAL *Journal*

notes

notes

_____

_____

_____

_____

_____

_____

_____

_____

_____

_____

_____

notes

_____

_____

_____

_____

_____

_____

_____

_____

_____

_____

_____

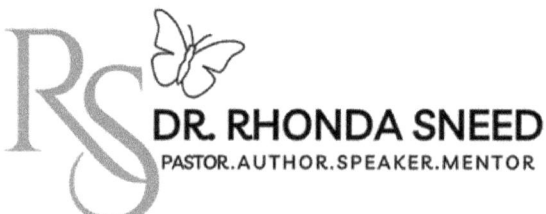

DR. RHONDA SNEED
PASTOR.AUTHOR.SPEAKER.MENTOR

(318) 597-2901
Rhonda.sneed@att.net
http://www.restoringsouls.org

Social Media
@Drrhondasneed

www.ingramcontent.com/pod-product-compliance
Lightning Source LLC
Chambersburg PA
CBHW051208120626
46547CB00013B/1254